MEDICAL BOARDS STEP 2
made ridiculously simple

Andreas Carl, M.D., Ph.D.
Adjunct Assistant Professor
University of Nevada School of Medicine
Department of Physiology and Cell Biology
Reno, NV 89557-0046

MedMaster, Inc., Miami

Diagnostic descriptions and criteria of psychiatric diseases have been adapted from the *Diagnostics and Statistical Manual of Mental Disorders*, Fourth edition (DSM IV) with permission of the American Psychiatric Association.

ISBN # 0-940780-55-0
Made in the United States of America

Published by
MedMaster, Inc.
P.O. Box 640028
Miami, FL 33164

For Manfred, Rosi, Olaf and Astrid

In Medical Practice You Encounter
Uncommon Presentations Of Common Diseases.

On The Medical Board Exams You Encounter
Common Presentations Of Uncommon Diseases.

PREFACE TO THE 3rd EDITION

With the new computerized testing, it is more important than ever to be able to recognize a case presentation (clinical vignette), formulate a differential diagnosis and be aware of management options. I have carefully revised all items and placed each chart into a context. Hopefully, this will make *"Medical Boards Made Ridiculously Simple"* much more useful as a study tool, in addition to being a great "memory aid". The management sections at the end of each chapter have been updated to reflect the current state of medical practice.

WHY THE CHART FORMAT?

Well, I made these charts for myself when I took the USMLE and found it a fantastic memory-aid! Charts allow a more logical arrangement of basic science facts that can easily be build upon rather than just a random collection of materials. Studying in such systematic fashion lets you avoid the "high-yield trap". I have chosen the chart-format in order to provide the maximum amount of information with the minimum amount of words. By concentrating on key associations you will certainly improve your performance in multiple choice situations.

WHAT THIS BOOK IS NOT:

This book is not meant as a "Mini-Harrison" of Medicine. *Medical Boards Step 2 Made Ridiculously Simple* has been designed as a **"last minute review"** so that you will have the key facts required to pass the USMLE Step 2 exam ready at hand.

I have written this book in a way to help you in the **decision making process**. For example, rather than listing all possible signs and symptoms of pulmonary embolism, you will find how to distinguish pulmonary embolism from myocardial infarction in a clinical setting. This has been accomplished by listing only the most important and most specific items in chart format, allowing you to rapidly compare similar or easily confused diagnoses. I believe that this approach will be most helpful - both in multiple choice situations and when seeing real patients!

HOW TO USE THIS BOOK?

This book is best used side by side with your other text and review books. You can "personalize" the charts by adding information that appears important or interesting to you. **The logical arrangement of medical facts in charts will make it possible to review all USMLE subjects just a few days before the exam**. I recommend reviewing the tables many times until they become boring. This is a good sign - meaning you recognize the stuff. It's not necessary to be able to actively reproduce all material given here, as long as you recognize the key associations in a "multiple choice situation".

> ➤ Use it during your course work to organize your thoughts
> ➤ Use it as a refresher course
> ➤ Use it as a last minute review

Most chapters of *Medical Boards Step 2 Made Ridiculously Simple* have two parts: A **Differential Diagnostics** section presented in chart format followed by a patient management section covering diseases listed by the National Board of Medical Examiners. You will find that many items on the USMLE Step 2 give patient data (history, symptoms and lab data) followed by the question "*what is the next most appropriate step in patient management*?" The **Patient Management** section of each chapter addresses just this question - what to do next ?!

While some may view the separation of diagnosis and management as somewhat artificial, I believe that it will make it easier for you to learn the essentials in the shortest possible time. Also keep in mind that diagnosis and management are different physician tasks and that you will actually receive two separate scores for these on your USMLE Step 2 exam.

Additional chapters of this book are: (1.) **Public Health** issues, do not skip this – the USMLE recognizes the importance of disease prevention! (2.) A list of **Signs and Symptoms** and (3.) an overview of commonly used **Diagnostic Tests** including their indications and interpretations. Since you are not required to know specific surgical techniques, I have included all **surgical topics** along with the other disciplines. Indications for surgery are given in the management sections.

How you score on the USMLE Step 2 exam not only depends on how hard you study, but also on what you study. Obviously, if you study what they ask, you will achieve a very high score. I have prepared this manuscript in order to help you maximize your efforts. The material has been selected based on my experience with medical exams in Germany and my more recent experiences taking the USMLE Step 1 and USMLE Step 2 exams in the United States.

I have tried to write the book I wish I would have had when I studied for the USMLE Step 2 exam and I have included all the information I wish I would have known when I took this exam.

I like to thank Dr. Suat Yasar, Dr. Bouke de Jong and numerous medical students for their helpful suggestions and critical reading of this manuscript, Dr. Stephen Goldberg for his editorial help and Steve Goldberg for providing his lively illustrations. Good luck, and please let me know any comments or suggestions you may have for future editions.

Please visit my web-site to share your experiences with other students:

www.usmle.net

If you are about to take the exam or just took it, you can contact me via e-mail:

andreas@usmle.net

HOW DOES THE STEP 2 COMPARE TO THE STEP 3 EXAM?

After you pass the USMLE Step 2 exam and complete your first year of Residency Training, you want to take the **USMLE Step 3 exam**. Fortunately, you will find that the Step 3 exam is similar in style, content and level of difficulty to the Step 2 exam. I recommend *Medical Boards Step 2 Made Ridiculously Simple* as a quick refresher just prior to taking the Step 3 exam. *Medical Boards Step 3 Made Ridiculously Simple* **is the perfect companion to my** *Medical Boards Step 2 Made Ridiculously Simple* **book**. While the Step 2 book presents material in a "disease-oriented approach" centered around organ systems, the Step 3 book presents material in a more "patient-oriented approach".

The two books are designed to go "hand-in-hand" and complement each other. The Step 2 book will give you a solid foundation to pass the Step 2 exam and also would serve you well for the Step 3. My *Medical Boards Step 3 Made Ridiculously Simple* extends the material in areas that are emphasized on the USMLE Step 3 exam, namely diagnostic approaches and patient management. **You will find** *Medical Boards Step 3 Made Ridiculously Simple* **also useful for a more in depth review of patient management for the Step 2 exam!**

All areas of Medicine are covered in both books, however the emphasis is different:

STEP 2 book	STEP 3 book
• Diseases and Organ Systems	• Diagnosis, Step-by-Step • Patient Management

vi

STUDY HINTS

There are three areas from the USMLE Step 1 that you will need to review:

STEP 1 book	
Pathology	- disease entities and mechanisms of disease
Microbiology	- infectious diseases
Pharmacology	- drug indications, side effects and contraindications

These topics are covered in detail in my book *Medical Boards Step 1 Made Ridiculously Simple*. In order to avoid repetition and to keep the present book as compact as possible **I have not repeated this information here**. I strongly advise you to spend at least one day each reviewing these areas.

BOOKS / MULTIPLE CHOICE QUESTIONS

Many excellent books are on the market, and you should have no difficulty choosing the right one for your personal learning style. It is usually better to know one book really well than to know a little of many books. I prefer the medium size text books, for example "*Cecil Essentials of Medicine*" (1) or "*Rudolph's Fundamentals of Pediatrics*" (17) over the somewhat shorter "pure review books" (Oklahoma Notes or NMS series). The extra material will improve your understanding and medical judgment and they are easier to read too.

You should practice at least a few hundred multiple choice questions under "real time" conditions before the actual exam. I particularly recommend the *National Medical Series Review for the USMLE Step 2* (14). These are most similar in style and difficulty to the real exam. Mark all the ones you got wrong and concentrate your studies on these areas. I made myself "error sheets" listing all my mistakes in single line statements. The day before the exam I read this list of facts I should have known to give me a last minute extra boost. It worked!

MEDICINE

The current political emphasis on primary care and family practice is reflected in the content of the USMLE Step 2. You would be very well advised to use any of the primary care medicine books for your preparation. **I especially recommend "*Medicine: A Primary Care Approach*"** (13). If you have somewhat limited time and want to read only one book - this is it. It is divided into 127 short chapters dealing with the common medical problems, each preceded by a case history.

PREVENTIVE MEDICINE / PUBLIC HEALTH

This often-underestimated topic is a very important part of the Medical Boards. You should know the risk factors of most cancers and leading causes of death. You should know immunization schedules for both children and adults. You should know when to do screening tests, and when not to do screening tests. Very detailed information can be found in my *Medical Boards Step 3 Made Ridiculously Simple* book.

SURGERY

No knowledge of any special surgical techniques is required - but you should know the difference between a Billroth-I and Billroth-II. Learn all you can about automobile accidents, the different types of injuries (blunt versus perforating trauma) associated with them and their treatment. It's a favorite topic.

OB/GYN

High yield topics: Normal development (puberty and menopause), menstrual cycle, infertility, differential diagnosis of bleeding during pregnancy, management of medical complications during pregnancy. Try to memorize major drugs that are contraindicated during pregnancy, and those which are allowed. *Obstetrics and Gynecology* by W.W. Beck (15) is my favorite from the NMS series - an easy to digest book covering the essentials.

PEDIATRICS

Despite what they say about children not being "little adults", there is significant overlap with internal medicine. If you choose to read a full book like *"Rudolph's Fundamentals of Pediatrics"* (17) you may want to concentrate on just a few chapters like neonatology, congenital defects, transmission of STDs during pregnancy and/or labor, nutrition, normal development and endocrine diseases.

PSYCHIATRY

Really all you need to know are the diagnostic definitions published in *"Quick Reference Guide to the DSM IV"* (16). If you have difficulty applying these somewhat abstract concepts to real cases you may want to read a few chapters in the *"DSM IV - Casebook"* (7). Remember: Biological psychiatry and drug treatment is "in." Psychoanalysis is "out."

TEST TAKING STRATEGIES

Many questions are extraordinarily long. I recommend to read the last sentence of a long question first, then take a quick glance at the answers. This way you know what they want before you endeavor to work your way through the patient's history and lab-data.

If you can't even guess a question, choose either the longest answer or the one that is most similar to other choices. Then move on. Watch your time - it's critical !

ADVICE FOR FOREIGN MEDICAL GRADUATES

Most US students take the USMLE Step2 after applying for a Residency position. As an IMG you do not have this luxury and you should take this exam very seriously. With the recent changes in health care policy it has become more and more difficult to find residency positions. Your score on the USMLE Step 2 may very well determine what kind of residency position you will get or if you "get in" at all. Your goal should not be to "just pass it," but to achieve an above average score and you should prepare yourself accordingly.

- Practice as many multiple choice questions as you can and practice at least a few hundred under real time conditions (stop watch).

- Learn patient management as thoroughly as possible, especially if you are from a country where health care delivery and the spectrum of diseases differ from the US.

- If you can, take advantage of morning or noon conferences at your local University Hospital.

www.usmle.net
➤ latest trends on the USMLE
➤ bulletin board
➤ book recommendations

ix

REFERENCES

1. Cecil Essentials of Medicine, W.B. Saunders Co.
2. Cecil Textbook of Medicine, W.B. Saunders Co.
3. Current Medical Diagnosis&Treatment, Appleton&Lange
4. Current Emergency Diagnosis&Treatment, Appleton&Lange
5. Current Obstetric&Gynecologic Diagnosis&Treatment, Appleton&Lange
6. Current Pediatric Diagnosis&Treatment, Appleton&Lange
7. Diagnostics and Statistical Manual of Mental Disorders, American Psychiatric Press
8. DSM IV Casebook, American Psychiatric Press
9. Harrison's Principles of Internal Medicine, McGraw-Hill
10. Internal Medicine, Ed. J.H. Stein, Mosby
11. Internal Medicine Pearls, Mosby-Yearbook
12. Mayo Internal Medicine Board Review, Mayo Foundation
13. Medicine: A Primary Care Approach, W.B. Saunders Co.
14. National Medical Series Review for the USMLE Step 2, Williams&Wilkins
15. Obstetrics and Gynecology, NMS series, Harwal Publishing
16. Quick Reference to the Diagnostic Criteria from DSM IV, Am. Psychiatric Press
17. Rudolph's Fundamentals of Pediatrics, Appleton&Lange
18. Rudolph's Pediatrics, Appleton&Lange
19. Synopsis of Psychiatry, Williams&Wilkins

CROSCROSCROSCROSCROSCROSCROSCROSCROSCRO

CONTENTS

TABLE OF CONTENTS

PUBLIC HEALTH ISSUES

SIGNS AND SYMPTOMS

DIAGNOSTIC TESTS

CARDIOVASCULAR DISEASES

RESPIRATORY DISEASES

GASTROINTESTINAL DISEASES

UROGENITAL DISEASES

SEXUALLY TRANSMITTED DISEASES

INFECTIOUS DISEASES

HEMATOLOGY

GYNECOLOGY

OBSTETRICS

PEDIATRICS

PUBLIC HEALTH ISSUES

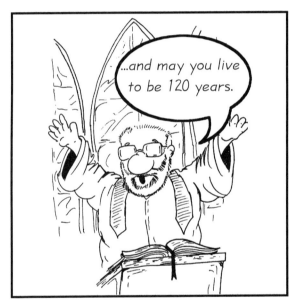

**The leading cause of death in people age 120...
curses.**

Part A: Epidemiology

1.1.) POPULATION DATA

Some definitions you need to know:

birth rate	live births / population
fertility rate	live births / females age 15 to 45
death rate	deaths / population
miscarriage	fetal death within first 20 weeks
stillbirth	fetal death at 28 weeks or later
neonatal mortality rate	deaths (<28 days) / live births
perinatal mortality rate	stillbirths + deaths (< 7 days) / total births
infant mortality rate	deaths (<1 year) / live births
maternal mortality rate	pregnancy-related deaths / live births

Rates are reported per 1,000 population per year except maternal mortality per 100,000 per year.

2

1.2.) <u>LEADING CAUSES OF DEATH</u>

neonates	• prematurity o congenital abnormalities
infants	• congenital abnormalities o injuries
teenagers, young adults	• motor vehicle accidents [1] • homicide o suicide
adults > 40 years	• heart disease o lung cancer o cerebrovascular disease
elderly	• heart disease o cerebrovascular disease o lung disease
death due to drug overdose	o tricyclic antidepressants

[1] ***Homicide is the leading cause of death in black teenagers.***
Suicide and accidents are more common in white teenagers.

1.3.) <u>SEX</u>

Diseases that are more common in males or females:

MALES	FEMALES
• coronary artery disease • cardiomyopathy	• mitral valve prolapse
• endangiitis obliterans • periarteritis nodosa	• Raynaud's phenomenon
• alcoholic cirrhosis • hemochromatosis	• primary biliary cirrhosis
• ankylosing spondylitis • Reiter's syndrome	• lupus erythematodes • scleroderma • arthrosis of finger joints
• COPD, lung carcinoma etc.	• endocrine diseases
• gout • porphyria • chronic lymphocytic leukemia • hairy cell leukemia	• anorexia nervosa

1.4.) ETHNICITY

Diseases that are more common in certain ethnic groups:

Caucasians	• cystic fibrosis
Mediterraneans	• β-thalassemia • G6PD deficiency
African Americans	• hemoglobinopathies (HbS, HbC) • α-thalassemia, β-thalassemia • G6PD deficiency • hypertension • homicide
Eskimos	• pseudocholinesterase deficiency
Ashkenazi Jews	• Gaucher's • Niemann-Pick • Tay-Sachs

1.5.) <u>OCCUPATION</u>

Diseases that are more common in certain professions:

abattoir workers	• brucellosis
bakery	• flour, fungi, dust (asthma)
battery manufacture or repair	• lead poisoning • cadmium poisoning
cotton industry	• byssinosis
dentists	• mercury
farmers	• pesticides • actinomycosis • brucellosis • erysipeloid • alveolitis
gardeners	• sporotrichosis
glass and ceramics industry	• silicosis, lead poisoning
insulation industry and ship building	• asbestosis • mesothelioma
mining	• dust, coal, silica
painters	• solvents • lead poisoning
radiator repair	• lead poisoning
rubber industry	• aromatic amines (bladder carcinoma)

1.6.) GEOGRAPHY

Diseases that are more common in certain areas of the US:

coccidioidomycosis	• Southwestern United States
histoplasmosis	• Ohio/Mississippi river
Lyme disease	• East Coast and Midwest of USA • Scandinavia
Rocky Mountain spotted fever	• East Coast of the USA (not Rocky Mountains!)
Western equine encephalitis	• West of Mississippi
Eastern equine encephalitis	• Atlantic and Gulf states
California encephalitis	• North-Central States of USA

1.7.) <u>ANIMALS</u>

Diseases that are transmitted by animals and insects:

__pasteurella__	• cat bites, dog bites
__anthrax__	• cattle, swine, wool
__brucellosis__	• cattle (dairy products) • goats (dairy products) • pigs
__Hanta virus__	• deer mice
__toxoplasmosis__	• cat feces
__psittacosis__	• birds
__leptospirosis__	• rats, dogs, cats
__Rocky Mountain spotted fever__ (*Rickettsia rickettsii*)	• dogs, rodents → ticks → humans
__epidemic typhus__ (*Rickettsia prowazekii*)	• humans → lice → humans
__endemic typhus__ (*Rickettsia typhi*)	• rodents → fleas → humans
__tularemia__	• rabbits → ticks → humans
__Lyme disease__ (*Borrelia burgdorferi*)	• mice → ticks → humans
__plague__ (*Yersinia pestis*)	• squirrels, rats
__Chagas' disease__ (*Trypanosoma*)	• kissing bug
__kala-azar__ (*Leishmania*)	• sandfly

1.8.) <u>RISK AND ODDS</u>

	DISEASE PRESENT	DISEASE ABSENT
risk factor present	A	B
risk factor absent	C	D

- **risk**   : A / (A+B)
- **odds**   : A / B

- **risk ratio**   : [A / (A+B)] / [C / (C+D)]
- **odds ratio**: [A / B] / [C / D]

- **attributable risk**   : risk $_{exposed}$ - risk $_{unexposed}$
- **relative risk (risk ratio)** : risk $_{exposed}$ / risk $_{unexposed}$

If risk is small (A << B), risk and odds will be almost the same.

- **Risk ratio** *can be determined from prospective* **cohort study**.
- *Risk ratio* <u>can not</u> *be determined from case-control study.*

- **Odds ratio** *can be determined from* **case-control study**.
- *If risk is low, odds ratio will give a good estimate of risk ratio.*

<u>Type I error</u>:
To claim a difference between groups when there is not (α).
<u>Type II error</u>:
To see no difference between groups when there is one (β).

Power: 1 - β

Part B: Preventive Medicine

1.9.) TYPES OF PREVENTION

primary prevention	**intervention before disease is present** ○ vaccinations ○ prevention of nutritional deficiencies ○ prevention of specific injuries
secondary prevention	**intervention during latent disease** ○ early detection of disease ○ screening
tertiary prevention	**intervention during symptomatic disease** ○ limitation of physical and social consequences of disease ○ rehabilitation

1.10.) <u>CORONARY HEART DISEASE</u>

Coronary heart disease is the leading cause of death in the US in both men and women. Preventive measures aim at reducing modifiable risk factors:

fixed risk factors	modifiable risk factors
• male sex • family history • older age	• cigarette smoking • high LDL • low HDL • diabetes mellitus • hypertension

 Cessation of smoking decreases most excess risk within 1 year.

 Reducing risk factors...
(1.) *slows progression of coronary disease.*
(2.) *may result in a disease regression in some patients.*
(3.) *significantly reduces coronary events.*

1.11.) <u>PULMONARY DISEASE</u>

Examples of preventive measures in lung diseases:

	PREVENTIVE MEASURES
primary prevention	• avoid environmental exposure • avoid occupational exposure • stop smoking
secondary prevention	• **Example: PPD screening** indications: - close contacts of persons with tuberculosis - immigrants from Africa, Asia, South America - residents of nursing homes - HIV positive persons
tertiary prevention	• **Example: COPD** - monitor blood oxygen saturation - give supplemental oxygen to prolong life

*Screening otherwise asymptomatic cigarette smokers for lung cancer (e.g. chest x-ray or sputum cytology) does not improve overall survival and is **not recommended**.*

1.12.) <u>OSTEOPOROSIS</u>

A) <u>FACTORS THAT DETERMINE BONE MINERALIZATION</u>:

ENHANCED	REDUCED
• estrogen	• glucocorticoids
• testosterone	• parathyroid hormone
• calcium	• thyroid hormone
• vit. D	
• weight bearing exercise	• renal failure

B) <u>TWO TYPES OF OSTEOPOROSIS</u>:

TYPE I ("postmenopausal")	TYPE II ("senile")
• affects only women	• affects men and women
• develops rapidly	• develops more gradually
• loss of trabecular bone (vertebrae, forearm)	• trabecular and cortical bone (femoral neck, tibia, pelvis)

➢ Bone loss is most rapid during first 5 years post menopause.
➢ Bone loss resumes if estrogen replacement is discontinued.
➢ Up to 30% of bone is lost before detectable by x-ray.
➢ DEXA scan preferred over CT or photon absorptiometry.

➢ Testosterone may be useful for men with gonadal deficiency.

1.13.) <u>PREGNANCY SCREENING</u>

hypertension	• monitor throughout pregnancy (weight gain, edema, blood pressure)
Rh incompatibility	• determine at first prenatal visit
rubella titer	• determine at first prenatal visit
sexually transmitted diseases	<u>screen at first prenatal visit:</u> o gonorrhea o syphilis o chlamydia o HBsAg o offer HIV
bacteriuria	• urine culture at first prenatal visit • treat bacteriuria, even if asymptomatic
triple screen [1]	• at 16-18 weeks
oral glucose tolerance	• at 24-28 weeks
amniocentesis	• consider for women > 35

[1] α-FP , hCG , estriol

1.14.) <u>NEONATAL SCREENING</u>

	MANDATORY FOR:
phenylketonuria	• all infants at birth
hypothyroidism	• all infants at birth
hemoglobin electrophoresis	• Africans • Mediterraneans • South East Asians

1.15.) <u>RHESUS FACTOR</u>

- **if unsensitized Rh- mother with Rh+ (or unknown) father:**
  give immunoglobulins at 25-30 weeks gestation.

- **if unsensitized Rh- mother delivers Rh+ infant:**
  give second dose of immunoglobulins within 72 hours after delivery.

1.16.) <u>IMMUNIZATIONS FOR INFANTS</u>

	birth	2m	4m	6m	15m	4-6y
hepatitis B	⬤	⬤		⬤		
haemophilus influenzae		⬤	⬤	⬤	⬤	
oral polio		⬤	⬤		⬤	⬤
DTP, DTaP		⬤	⬤	⬤	⬭	⬭
MMR					⬤	⬤

 If mother positive for HBsAg also give immunoglobulins to newborn.

Oral Polio (Sabin):	- live-attenuated - lifelong immunity - local gut and systemic immunity - may cause paralytic disease
Injectable Polio (Salk):	- inactivated - requires booster every 4-5 years - minimal gut immunity - no risk of paralytic disease

1.17.) __IMMUNIZATIONS FOR ADULTS__

dT	• every 10 years
measles	• if born before 1957 : assume "natural" immunity • if born after 1957 : recommend 2 doses • protective if given within 72 h of exposure • pregnant or immune compromised : give IgG
Pneumovax (give once)	• elderly > 65 years • chronic ill persons: COPD, HIV, CHF, DM etc. • prior to splenectomy
influenza (every autumn)	• elderly > 65 years • chronic ill persons: COPD, HIV, CHF, DM etc. • contacts and health care personnel

 No live vaccines for HIV positive infants or adults __except MMR__ !

1.18.) <u>IMMUNIZATION REACTIONS</u>

It is important to anticipate reactions to vaccines:

IF PRESENT:	AVOID:
allergy to egg	<ul><li>MMR</li><li>influenza</li></ul>
allergy to neomycin	<ul><li>MMR</li><li>oral polio</li></ul>
immunodeficiency	<ul><li>MMR (but is o.k. for HIV+ patients)</li><li>oral polio</li></ul>
neurologic disorder	<ul><li>DTP</li></ul>

1.19.) TETANUS PROPHYLAXIS

MANAGEMENT OF TETANUS-PRONE WOUNDS:

Immunization History	Tetanus Toxoid	Anti-Tetanus Immune Globulin
3 prior doses		
• clean minor wound	yes if > 10 years	no
• other wound	yes if > 5 years	no
immunization unknown or less than 3 doses		
• clean minor wound	yes	no
• other wound	yes	yes

1.20.) <u>CANCER RISK FACTORS</u>

Many cancers can be avoided by following a healthy lifestyle:

lung cancer	• smoking • secondhand smoke • radiation (radon)
nasopharyngeal cancer	• smoking • alcohol
cervix cancer	• early age at first intercourse • multiple sex partners
breast cancer	• no or late pregnancies • obesity • high fat diet • radiation (mammography ?)
liver cancer	• hepatitis B or C infection • vinyl chloride
colon/rectum cancer	• diet high in saturated fat • diet low in fruits, vegetable, fiber
bladder cancer	• aromatic amines
skin cancer	• sun light (UV-B radiation)

<u>**Cigarette smoking also increases the risk of:**</u>
(1.) cervix cancer
(2.) bladder cancer
(3.) pancreas cancer

1.21.) CANCER SCREENING

A) SCREENING TESTS THAT ARE RECOMMENDED:

breast cancer	> **40 years:** annual clinical exam > **50 years:** mammography every 1-2 years
cervix cancer	• Pap smears every 1-3 years • for all women who are or have been sexually active
prostate cancer	> 40 years : **digital rectal exam** • routine PSA screening not recommended
colon cancer	• fecal occult blood if > 50 years or family history • **colonoscopy if family history of polyposis**
testicular cancer	• if history of **cryptorchidism or testicular atrophy**

B) SCREENING TESTS THAT ARE NOT RECOMMENDED:

ovarian cancer	• routine screening **not recommended**
endometrial cancer	• routine screening **not recommended** • watch for abnormal uterine bleeding in elderly women
lung cancer	• routine screening **not recommended**

1.22.) <u>SOCIAL INSURANCE</u>

MEDICARE	MEDICAID
• part of Social Security Trust Fund • federally administered	• paid from general tax revenue • administered by the States
• for people > 65 years • for people who receive social security benefits due to disability	• for poor people (usually on welfare)
• covers some home care • covers some nursing home care • covers most but not all hospitalization	• pays medical care expenses • pays long-term nursing home care after personal resources have been exhausted

 "Care for the elderly and aid the poor"

22

Part C: Drug Abuse

1.23.) ABUSE & DEPENDENCE

DEFINITIONS:

ABUSE	DEPENDENCE
recurrent substance use resulting in:	recurrent substance use resulting in:
<ul><li>failure to fulfill obligations</li><li>dangerous situations (e.g. DUI)</li><li>social difficulties</li><li>legal difficulties</li></ul>	<ul><li>**tolerance***</li><li>**withdrawal syndromes***</li><li>unsuccessful efforts to quit</li><li>preoccupation with obtaining drug resulting in loss of social, occupational or recreational activities.</li></ul>

* indicates physiological dependence

- Almost all drugs can cause delirium during intoxication.

- Withdrawal delirium is only common with alcohol, sedatives and anxiolytic drugs.

23

1.24.) ALCOHOL AND SEDATIVES

INTOXICATION	WITHDRAWAL
<ul><li>slurred speech</li><li>unsteady gait</li><li>incoordination</li><li>nystagmus</li></ul>	**"uncomplicated"** [1] **6-8 hours after cessation**<ul><li>autonomic hyperactivity</li><li>seizures</li><li>hand tremor</li><li>insomnia</li><li>nausea, vomiting</li></ul>**perceptual disturbances** **8-12 hours after cessation**<ul><li>delusions, hallucinations</li></ul>**delirium tremens** **72 hours after cessation**<ul><li>agitation, unpredictable behavior</li><li>lost reality testing</li><li>mortality 20% if untreated</li></ul>

[1] *even uncomplicated (i.e. no delirium) withdrawal may be life threatening!*

PERCEPTUAL DISTURBANCE:
Hallucinations and illusions with intact reality testing, i.e. the patient knows that these are due to disease rather than external reality.

DRUG-INDUCED PSYCHOTIC DISORDER:
Hallucinations and illusions, patient loses reality testing.

1.25.) __CANNABIS__

INTOXICATION	WITHDRAWAL
• euphoria • anxiety • sensation of slowed time • social withdrawal • **conjunctival injection** • dry mouth • increased appetite	• none

1.26.) __LSD__

INTOXICATION	WITHDRAWAL
• marked anxiety • paranoid ideas • fear of losing one's mind • **pupillary dilation** • tachycardia • sweating • tremors	• none • **flashbacks:** • re-experiencing hallucinations and illusions after cessation of drug use

1.27.) <u>AMPHETAMINES / COCAINE</u>

INTOXICATION	WITHDRAWAL
• euphoria • vigilance • anxiety, tension • **pupillary dilation** • tachycardia or bradycardia • psychomotor agitation or retardation • weight loss	• dysphoria • fatigue • unpleasant dreams

1.28.) OPIOIDS

INTOXICATION	WITHDRAWAL
• initial euphoria • then apathy • **pupillary constriction** • slurred speech • drowsiness, coma	• **severe, but not life threatening** • dysphoria • nausea, vomiting, diarrhea • sweating, lacrimation • muscle aches, fever

1.29.) PHENCYCLIDINE

INTOXICATION	WITHDRAWAL
• aggressive, impulsive behavior • agitation • **horizontal and vertical nystagmus** • hypertension • ataxia • muscle rigidity • hyperacusis • seizures	• none, but psychosis may last for days or weeks following use of PCP

SIGNS AND SYMPTOMS

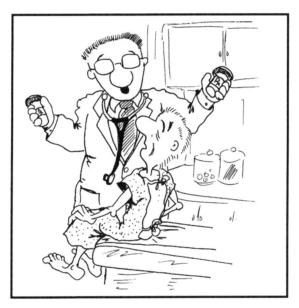

"The first drug is to control your high blood pressure.
The second drug is to counteract the *first drug's* side effects,
but can have its own side effect of *increasing* the blood
pressure. But not to worry. If that happens, simply take
more of the first medicine."

2.1.) <u>CARDIOVASCULAR SIGNS</u>

S3 gallop [1] (ventricular)	**dilated cardiomyopathy** • aortic insufficiency • congestive heart failure • volume overload
S4 gallop [2] (atrial)	**constrictive cardiomyopathy (stiff ventricle)** • arterial hypertension • myocardial ischemia or infarction • AV block
pulsus paradoxus	**exaggerated decline of BP during inspiration** • cardiac tamponade • constrictive pericarditis • massive pulmonary embolism
pulsus alternans	**beat to beat change in pulse amplitude** • indicates left ventricular failure
orthopnea	**difficulty breathing in supine position** (increased hydrostatic pressure in pulmonary circulation) • COPD • left ventricular failure
Kussmaul's sign	**distention of jugular veins with inspiration** • constrictive pericarditis

[1] *may be normal in children and young adults*
[2] *may be normal in athletes*

2.2) <u>RESPIRATORY SIGNS</u>

Biot	<ul><li>breaths of equal volume alternating with episodes of apnea</li><li>a/w central cerebral lesions</li></ul>
Cheyne Stokes	<ul><li>waxing and waning (hyperpnea ↔ apnea)</li><li>common at high altitude</li><li>a/w increased intracranial pressure</li></ul>
Kussmaul	<ul><li>hyperventilation (deep, rapid, sighing)</li><li>a/w metabolic acidosis</li></ul>
barrel chest	<ul><li>increased ant./post. diameter of chest</li><li>late sign of COPD</li><li>due to loss of lung elasticity</li></ul>
breath odors	**fruity:** ketoacidosis **sweet, musty:** liver failure **uriniferous:** uremia, renal failure **foul:** lung abscess, bronchiectasis
nasal flaring	<ul><li>respiratory distress</li><li>important sign in children who can't tell !</li></ul>

2.3.) <u>AUSCULTATION</u>

crackles (rales, crepitations)	• rattling noises, usually during inspiration • movement of air through fluid-filled airways • **bronchitis, pneumonia, lung edema**
rhonchi	• continuous, resembles deep snore • narrowing of large airways • **aspiration, bronchospasm**
wheezing	• rhonchi with high-pitched musical quality • cannot be cleared by coughing • **bronchospasm, mucosal edema, asthma**
stridor	• loud, musical sound • usually inspiratory (may be expiratory in severe cases) • **obstruction of larynx or trachea** • may indicate life threatening narrowing of airways, especially in children

2.4.) <u>EYES AND EARS</u>

scotoma	**areas of partial blindness** • glaucoma • chorioretinitis • macular degeneration • migraine (scintillating scotomas)
arcus senilis	**green-white, opaque ring at corneal periphery** • fat deposits
Horner's syndrome	**damage to cervical chain ganglia resulting in:** • pupil constriction • ptosis (eye lid drooping) • warm, dry facial skin
hearing loss	**conductive hearing loss** [1] • cerumen • tympanic membrane perforation • otitis media • otosclerosis **sensorineural hearing loss** [2] • presbyacusis • ototoxic drugs • Ménière's • acoustic neurinoma
tinnitus	**ear ringing** • acoustic neurinoma • labyrinthitis • Ménière's disease • small tympanic membrane perforations • hypertension • salicylates, quinine, aminoglycosides

[1] *Weber lateralizes towards sick ear.*
[2] *Weber lateralizes towards healthy ear.*

2.5.) <u>SIGNS OF INFECTION</u>

Brudzinski's sign	**meningeal irritation** • flexion of hips and knees in response to passive flexion of neck
Kernig's sign	**meningeal irritation** • hamstring muscle pain when examiner lifts the supine patient's extended leg
opisthotonus	**meningeal irritation** • severe muscle spasm causing back arch • more common in infants
McBurney's sign	**appendicitis** • rebound tenderness at McBurney's point (1/3 from ant. sup. spine to umbilicus)
Murphy's sign	**acute cholecystitis** • arrest of inspiration when palpating liver
Koplik's spots	**measles** • small red spots with bluish-white center on buccal mucosa • generalized rash will follow in 1-2 days
Janeway spots [1]	**infective endocarditis** • tiny red lesions on palms and soles
Roth spots [1]	**infective endocarditis** • subretinal hemorrhages with pale center
Osler's nodes [1]	**infective endocarditis** • tender, raised nodules on finger pads and toes

[1] *these "famous signs" are actually not very common.*

2.6.) <u>ARTHRITIS</u>

Examine patients for Heberden's nodes, swan neck deformity and tophi:

osteoarthritis	**Heberden's nodes** • painless bony enlargement of DIP
rheumatoid arthritis	**swan neck deformity** • hyperextended PIP • slightly flexed DIP <u>also</u>: • volar subluxation of MCP • ulnar deviation of fingers
gout	**tophi** • painless, nodular swelling (uric acid deposits) • ears, hands, feet

2.7.) <u>MALIGNANCIES</u>

Important signs that should alert you to malignancies:

Virchow's node	• palpable supraclavicular lymph node • a/w stomach cancer
Pancoast's	• shoulder pain (brachial plexus) • Horner's syndrome (cervical chain ganglia) • a/w apical lung tumors
Eaton-Lambert	• myasthenia • a/w small cell carcinoma (lung)
Trousseau's	• migratory thrombophlebitis • a/w adenocarcinomas: breast, lung, prostate...
peau d'orange	• edematous thickening of breast skin • a/w breast cancer (late sign)

2.8.) TRAUMA

Battle's sign [1]	**basilar skull fracture** • ecchymosis over mastoid • develops 24-36h after trauma
Raccoon's eyes [1]	**basilar skull fracture** • bilateral periorbital ecchymosis
Cullen's sign	**intra-abdominal bleeding** • hemorrhagic patches around umbilicus
Turner's sign	**intra-abdominal bleeding** • hemorrhagic patches at flanks
anterior drawer sign	• anterior cruciate ligament
posterior drawer sign	• posterior cruciate ligament
McMurray's sign	**meniscal tear** • "click" or "pop" elicited by lower leg manipulation

[1] *important signs since basilar skull fractures are easily missed on x-ray.*

2.9.) <u>MISCELLANEOUS SIGNS</u>

carpopedal spasm	• tetany, hypocalcemia
Trousseau's sign	• carpopedal spasm induced by inflating cuff on upper arm for several minutes
Chvostek's sign	• spasm of facial muscles elicited by tapping the patient's lower jaw area just anterior to earlobe
Homans' sign	• deep calf pain resulting from dorsiflexion of foot • indicates deep **venous thrombosis**
Nicoladoni's sign	• bradycardia when applying pressure to **arteriovenous fistula**
Ortolani's sign	• "click" upon abduction of a newborn's thigh • indicates **congenital hip dysplasia**
Rumpel-Leede sign	• place a tourniquet around upper arm and watch for distal petechiae • indicates severe **thrombocytopenia**
spider angioma	• a form of telangiectasia • most common on face and neck • characteristic for **liver cirrhosis**
pica	• **craving for inedible substances** • in children may indicate malnutrition, iron deficiency… • in adults usually indicates psychological disturbance

2.10.) <u>NERVE & MUSCLE</u>

asterixis	• "flapping tremor" • most commonly involves **wrist joint and fingers** • hallmark of hepatic encephalopathy • also seen in uremic syndrome
ataxia	• **incoordination of voluntary movements** • cerebellar • sensory (impaired proprioception)
athetosis	• **slow involuntary snakelike movements** • (especially face, neck and upper extremities) • due to damage of basal ganglia, • e.g. birth hypoxia, kernicterus • often combined with chorea
chorea	• **bursts of rapid, jerky movements** • may appear purposeful • **Huntington's:** chorea plus intellectual decline • **Wilson's disease:** chorea plus hemolytic anemia • sometimes caused by phenothiazines
cogwheel rigidity	• **jerking of arm muscles when passively stretched** • cardinal sign of Parkinson's • sometimes caused by antipsychotic drugs
dysdiadochokinesia	• difficulty performing rapidly alternating movements • **cerebellar disease**
Gower's sign	• sign of **proximal muscle weakness** (muscular dystrophy) • characteristic maneuver to rise from the floor
fasciculations	• minor muscle contractions (single motor units) • **do not cause joint movements** • normal in tense, anxious or tired persons • early sign of organophosphate poisoning

2.11.) <u>REFLEXES</u>

sucking reflex **palmar grasp reflex**	• weak in premature infants • fully developed after 36 weeks of gestation
tonic neck reflex	• turn face to one side (supine position): arms and leg on face side will extend • indicates neurological dysfunction if constantly present
Babinski reflex	• firmly stroke lateral sole of feet • dorsiflexion of great toe, fanning of other toes • **normal up to 2 years of age**
Moro reflex	• "startle reflex" • flexion of leg • embracing posture of arms • **normal up to 6 months of age**
automatic walking	• full-term newborns at 40 weeks tend to "walk" in heel-toe progression • preterm infants at 40 weeks tend to "walk" in toe-heel progression

 An asymmetric Moro reflex occurs with Erb's palsy (birth trauma).

2.12.) <u>BRAIN STEM SIGNS</u>

doll's eye sign	• **indicates brain stem dysfunction when absent** (i.e. eyes remain fixed in mid position when head is turned from side to side) • absent doll's eye sign is normal in neonates • don't do when cervical spine injury is suspected!
Argyll Robertson pupils	• small, irregular pupils • **respond to near accommodation** • **do not respond to light** • syphilis stage 3 (tabes dorsalis)
decorticate posture	• **legs extended, arms flexed** • damage to corticospinal tract • better prognosis than decerebrate
decerebrate posture	• **legs and arms extended** • damage to upper brainstem

2.13.) <u>PSYCHIATRIC SIGNS</u>

aphasia	• receptive[1] or expressive[2] language disorder
apraxia	• failure to do tasks, despite intact motor function
agnosia	• failure to recognize
dementia	• gradual impairment of cognitive functions, memory **Alzheimer dementia:** early memory loss **multi-infarct dementia:** steplike decline
delirium	• **acute, organic, short lasting** • clouded consciousness • confusion, disorientation, anxiety • sometimes hallucinations
delusions	• persistent false belief despite invalidating evidence • grandeur, paranoia • somatic delusions
illusions	• misperception of external stimuli
hallucinations	• perception without external stimuli

---

[1] **Wernicke:** - speech is fluent but rambling
             - patient has difficulty understanding spoken or written language

[2] **Broca:**   - word-finding difficulty resulting in non-fluent speech
             - little or no difficulty understanding spoken or written language

 Both Wernicke's and Broca's patients cannot repeat words or phrases.

DIAGNOSTIC TESTS

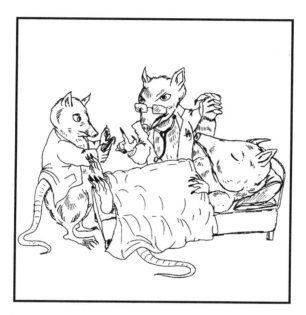

"Just drop his hand over his head. He doesn't want
to hurt himself. If it hits his head, he's comatose.
If it misses, he's playing possum."

3.1.) <u>MOLECULAR TESTS</u>

The USMLE recognizes the importance of molecular techniques for the medicine of the 21st Century and once obscure laboratory techniques have become mainstream. Here are some methods you should be very familiar with:

PCR	• **to amplify DNA fragments** o detection of viral DNA in serum (HIV: acute retroviral syndrome) o forensics (blood , semen) o detection and monitoring of cancer genes (p53, RAS etc...)
RT-PCR (reverse transcription)	• **to amplify RNA fragments** o analysis of gene expression
ELISA	• **to detect specific antigens or antibodies** o screening test for HIV antibodies o auto-antibodies o tumor markers o hormone assays
Southern Blot	• **detection of specific DNA sequences** o to detect gene mutations
Western Blot	• **detection of specific proteins** o HIV antibody pattern in patient's serum
RFLP	• **restriction endonucleases leave DNA fragments of various lengths** o DNA "fingerprinting" o paternity test o genomics: linkage of diseases to specific chromosomal regions

3.2.) <u>WATER AND SALT</u>

	MOST COMMON CAUSES:
hyponatremia high osmolarity	• hyperglycemia • use of hypertonic mannitol
hyponatremia normal osmolarity	• **hyperlipidemia** • **hyperproteinemia** (e.g. multiple myeloma)
hyponatremia low osmolarity	• SIADH • renal failure
hypernatremia [1] **ECV expanded**	• indicates **net Na$^+$ gain** • if mild: Cushing's or hyperaldosteronism • if severe: patient who received hypertonic saline
hypernatremia [1] **ECV depleted**	• **diarrhea, sweating, renal losses** • if patient is not thirsty, suspect hypothalamic tumor

[1] *always a/w hyperosmolarity!*

- Evaluate plasma Na$^+$ always in the context of osmolarity and ECV.

- Correct hypernatremia and hyponatremia very slowly (0.5 mM/hour).
  (danger of central pontine myelinolysis!)

3.3.) <u>POTASSIUM AND CALCIUM</u>

	MOST COMMON CAUSES:
hypokalemia	• **Hyperaldosteronism:** Conn (low renin) Bartter (high renin) • **loss:** renal (diuretics) diarrhea laxative abuse • **transcellular shift: alkalosis** acute glucose load insulin excess
hyperkalemia	• **Addison's** • **ACE inhibitors** o artifact: RBC hemolysis during blood drawing o rhabdomyolysis, tumor lysis o distal renal tubular acidosis • **transcellular shift: acidosis**
hypocalcemia	• **chronic renal failure** (phosphate retention) o lack of dietary Ca^{2+} and vit. D o hypoparathyroidism
hypercalcemia	• **bone cancer, metastases** o hyperparathyroidism o hypervitaminosis D

Free Ca^{2+} depends on pH;
acidosis → high free Ca^{2+}
alkalosis → low free Ca^{2+} (tetany)

3.4.) pH AND BLOOD GAS

simple hypoxia ($PaCO_2$ normal)	• ARDS • pneumonia
respiratory acidosis	• pH < 7.35; PaCO2 > 45 mmHg • COPD
metabolic acidosis	• pH < 7.35; HCO3 < 24 mEq/l • check anion gap! • ketoacidosis • renal failure • acute MI
respiratory alkalosis	• pH > 7.45; PaCO2 < 35 mmHg • anxiety, hysteria • pulmonary embolism • salicylate intoxication (early phase)
metabolic alkalosis	• pH > 7.45; HCO3 > 28 mEq/l • severe vomiting • gastric suction • hypokalemia

Anion gap = $[Na^+] - [Cl^- + HCO_3^-]$ = 8-12 mM/l

Normal anion gap: - diarrhea
                                  - renal tubular acidosis

Increased anion gap: - lactic acidosis
                                     - ketoacidosis
                                     - salicylates
                                     - alcohol (ethanol etc.)

3.5.) <u>LIVER & KIDNEYS</u>

AST (GOT)	• **hepatitis** • **acute MI:** detectable: 6-10 h • peak: 24-48h • **drugs:** antibiotics, oral contraceptives...
gamma-GT	• persistent liver cell damage • **alcoholism** • **drugs:** aminoglycosides, warfarin...
bilirubin	• **direct (conjugated):** biliary obstruction drug induced cholestasis Dubin-Johnson, Rotor's • **indirect (unconjugated):** hemolytic anemia physiologic jaundice of the newborn Gilbert's, Crigler-Najjar...
BUN	• **renal failure** • dehydration • high protein intake
creatinine [1]	• **renal failure** • diet: meat...
uric acid	• **gout** • leukemia, metastatic cancer chemotherapy! • food high in purines: brain, heart, kidneys, roe, sardines, scallops

[1] *creatinine <u>clearance</u> is more sensitive indicator of renal function (GFR).*

3.6.) <u>BLOOD LIPIDS</u>

cholesterol	TC = HDL + LDL + VLDL $\quad$ = HDL + LDL + triglycerides/5 TC $\;>$ 240 mg/dl : increased risk for CHD LDL > 160 mg/dl : increased risk for CHD HDL < 35 mg/dl : increased risk for CHD HDL > 60 mg/dl : considered "protective" LDL/HDL < 4 desirable
triglycerides	• levels increase with age • TG > 200 mg/dl: increased risk for CHD • estrogen and oral contraceptives increase triglycerides

<u>RULE OUT SECONDARY CAUSES OF HYPERLIPIDEMIA</u>:
(1.) diet: alcohol, saturated fats
(2.) drugs: steroids, thiazides, beta-blockers
(3.) diseases: diabetes, hypothyroidism, uremia

3.7.) <u>IRON</u>

Iron is the essential central atom in heme and cytochromes.

serum iron	**increase:** hemolysis hemochromatosis hemosiderosis **decrease:** anemia of chronic disease iron deficiency anemia blood loss
ferritin	**increase:** hemochromatosis hemosiderosis **decrease:** iron deficiency anemia
total iron binding capacity (=transferrin)	**increase:** blood loss iron deficiency anemia oral contraceptives! **decrease:** anemia of chronic disease cirrhosis nephrotic syndrome
transferrin saturation	**if < 15%** : iron deficiency anemia

3.8.) <u>ELECTROPHORESIS</u>

A) <u>SERUM</u>

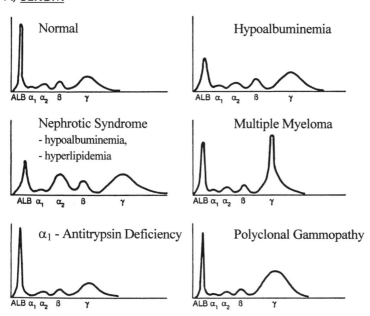

B) <u>URINE</u>

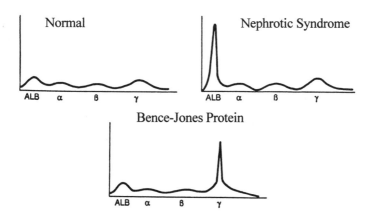

From *Clinician's Pocket Reference*, 8th edition, page 75, edited by L.G. Gomella.Appleton&Lange, 1997. Used with permission

3.9.) <u>IMAGING - 1</u>

chest x-ray (CXR)	• pneumonia • pneumonitis • neoplasms, metastases o not for routine screening for lung cancer!
expiratory CXR	• to visualize small pneumothorax
lateral decubitus CXR	• to visualize small pleural effusions
lung V/Q scan	• normal scan rules out pulmonary embolism
pulmonary angiography	• most accurate diagnostic procedure for embolism, but do only if V/Q scan is "non-diagnostic" • AV malformation
acute abdominal series (for initial evaluation)	• supine and upright, abdominal and CXR • watch for gas pattern, foreign bodies, renal and liver shadows, psoas shadow
barium enema	• indications: unresolved diarrhea, heme-pos. stools, change in bowel habits
air-contrast barium enema	• double contrast delineates mucosa • polyps, ulcerative colitis
ERCP	• visualizes common bile and pancreatic ducts • stones, obstructions, ductal pattern o may induce acute pancreatitis!

3.10.) <u>IMAGING - 2</u>

ultrasound	**B mode:** two-dimensional, fetal imaging **M mode:** measurement of cardiac chambers and movement of all 4 valves **Doppler:** to quantitate blood flow

IV pyelogram	• **pyelonephritis**
	  - small kidneys
	  - deformed calyces
	• **glomerulonephritis**
	  - kidneys and calyces look normal
	• **polycystic kidney**
	  - large kidney
	  - "spider" calyces

retrograde pyelogram	• if kidneys and ureters could not be visualized on IV pyelogram • can be done if patient is allergic to IV contrast
^{99m}Tc sulfur colloid scan	• detects GI bleeding
hepatobiliary scintigram	• 99mTc IDA • nonvisualization of gall bladder is diagnostic for obstruction of cystic duct (acute cholecystitis)
thallium scan	• myocardial perfusion • normal myocardium appears "hot" • **ischemic areas appear "cold"**
^{99m}TC pyrophosphate scan	• **recently damaged myocardium appears "hot"**

3.11.) <u>TOMOGRAPHY</u>

MRI	CT
MRI is better than CT for:	**CT is better than MRI for:**
• brain, spinal cord • soft tissues • renal masses	• subdural and epidural hematomas
Disadvantages:	Disadvantages:
• claustrophobia • longer scanning time • contraindicated if patient has metallic implants or pacemakers	• radiation exposure

3.12.) <u>CLASSIC X-RAY SIGNS</u>

Kerley's B lines	• congestive heart failure • lung edema
unilateral high diaphragm	• paralysis • atelectasis • abscess
coin lesions (lung)	• calcified granulomas • primary carcinoma • metastases
egg-shell calcifications (hilar lymph nodes)	• silicosis, sarcoidosis
ground glass appearance	• sarcoidosis, miliary tuberculosis • pneumoconiosis
honeycombing	• endstage lung fibrosis
water bottle	• pericardial effusion
beak-like	• esophagus achalasia
lead-pipe	• ulcerative colitis
cobble-stoning	• Crohn's disease
napkin-ring	• colon cancer (right side)
apple core	• colon cancer (left side)
cotton-wool skull	• Paget's disease
punched out radiolucent areas of skull	• multiple myeloma

CARDIOVASCULAR DISEASES

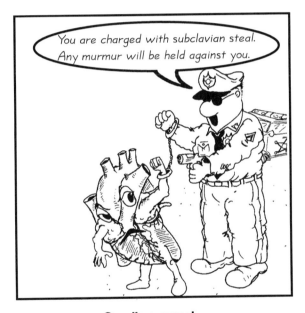

Cardiac arrest.

4.1.) ECG PATTERNS: ELECTROLYTES

Try to relate the ECG pattern to the 5 phases of the cardiac action potential to
understand the characteristic effects of electrolyte disorders:

hypokalemia	• **prolonged, flat T waves** • U waves	
hyperkalemia	• **tall, peaked T waves** • **widening of QRS**	
hypocalcemia	• **prolonged ST segment**	
hypercalcemia	• **shortened ST segment**	

digitalis	• **prolonged PR interval**
	  (watch for AV block)
	• **shortened QT interval**
	  (watch for ectopic systoles)
	• **deep, scooped ST**	

4.2.) <u>ECG PATTERNS: ISCHEMIA</u>

Both ST depression and ST elevation can be a sign of ischemia:

ST depression	• subendocardial ischemia
ST elevation	• transmural ischemia • coronary artery spasm
q waves	• transmural infarction
T wave inversion	• nonspecific finding • may be present after MI • transient T wave inversion is seen during ischemia

 A normal ECG does not exclude coronary artery disease or acute MI.

	ARTERIES	ABNORMALITIES	IN LEADS:
anteroseptal MI	LAD	V1 - V3	I, aVL
anterolateral MI	CRFLX	V4-V6	I, aVL
inferior MI	RCA		II, III, aVF
posterior MI	RCA	reciprocal V1 - V3	

4.3.) <u>ECG PATTERNS: ARRHYTHMIAS</u>

Ventricular arrhythmias are much more serious than atrial ones but easily recognized on ECG by their abnormal QRS complex. More subtle are arrhythmias due to abnormal conduction between the atria and ventricles:

AV block - 1 degree	• PR interval > 0.2 s
AV block - 2 degree	**Mobitz type I (Wenckebach)** • progressive lengthening of PR interval followed by QRS dropout
AV block - 2 degree	**Mobitz type II** • constant PR, sudden dropouts of QRS • Adam-Stokes syncope
AV block - 3 degree (complete)	• P waves independent of QRS • QRS wide if originating in ventricle
Wolff-Parkinson-White	• accessory AV pathway causing **pre-excitation** • may trigger reentrant tachyarrhythmias • short PR interval < 0.12 s • increased QRS > 0.12 s • delta waves (= slurred QRS): • a/w Ebstein's anomaly

4.4.) <u>PACEMAKERS</u>

You must memorize indications for pacemakers:

NOT INDICATED	INDICATED
• asymptomatic sick sinus syndrome • asymptomatic atrial fibrillation • first degree AV block • asymptomatic second degree AV block (Mobitz I)	• symptomatic second degree AV block (Mobitz I) • second degree block (Mobitz II) even if asymptomatic • third degree AV block

4.5.) <u>CARDIAC ENZYMES</u>

Cardiac muscle specific enzymes are sensitive and specific indicators to diagnose myocardial infarction:

CK (MB fraction)	• most sensitive and specific marker of MI • acute MI: **detectable at 6-12 h** peak at 12-20 h
LDH 1	• acute MI: **detectable at 12-24 h** peak in 2-5 days **LDH 1: cardiac, RBCs** LDH 2: cardiac, RBCs LDH 3: lung LDH 4: liver, skeletal muscle, kidney LDH 5: liver, skeletal muscle **LDH1 / LDH2 > 1 ("flipped"): indicates MI**

Negative creatine kinase MB at admission does not rule out MI.

20-30% of myocardial infarctions are "silent", i.e. do not cause pain. This is more common in diabetic patients.

4.6.) <u>CARDIAC CAUSES OF CHEST PAIN</u>

classic angina	<ul><li>substernal pain</li><li>transient (<10 min)</li><li>provoked by exercise</li><li>relieved by rest or nitrates</li><li>**ST depression**</li></ul>
unstable angina	<ul><li>change in pattern (more frequent, severe or prolonged)</li><li>angina at rest or at night</li><li>**ST depression**</li></ul>
variant angina (Prinzmetal's)	<ul><li>due to coronary artery vasospasm</li><li>not provoked by exercise!</li><li>**ST elevation**</li></ul>
myocardial infarction	<ul><li>substernal pain → arm, shoulder, jaw</li><li>lasts > 30 min</li><li>not relieved by rest or nitrates</li><li>**ST elevations, T inversions**</li></ul>
pericarditis	<ul><li>sharp chest pain</li><li>aggravated by deep breathing</li><li>pericardial friction rub</li><li>**non-specific ST elevations**</li></ul>
dissecting aortic aneurysm	<ul><li>"tearing" knifelike pain</li><li>sudden onset, long duration</li><li>may radiate to neck, chest or back</li></ul>

Patients with chest pain should undergo stress testing, unless contraindicated:

<u>Contraindications for stress testing:</u>
(1.) recent onset of unstable angina
(2.) uncontrolled hypertension
(3.) severe congestive heart failure

4.7.) <u>OTHER CAUSES OF CHEST PAIN</u>

While chest pain is always alarming to the patients, there are many causes other than cardiac ischemia:

pulmonary embolism	• sudden onset **dyspnea** / tachypnea • pleuritic chest pain • hemoptysis indicates pulmonary infarction
pneumothorax	• sudden onset sharp pain • aggravated by breathing • **hyperresonant** to percussion • absent tactile fremitus
pleurisy	• well localized pain • aggravated by breathing • **dull** to percussion
peptic ulcer	• burning, gnawing pain • lower substernal area, epigastrium • **relieved by antacids** or food
psychosomatic	• sharp, often localized to a point • usually of short duration

4.8.) <u>COMPLICATIONS OF MI</u>

arrhythmia	• dizziness, palpitations • syncope
congestive heart failure	• dyspnea, orthopnea • S3 gallop, S4 gallop • rales, wheezes (cardiac asthma) • cardiogenic shock
myocardial rupture	• tamponade, shock, death • typically **occurs with small infarcts!**
papillary muscle rupture	• hyperacute onset pulmonary edema • loud systolic murmur (mitral regurgitation)
septal rupture	• new onset holosystolic murmur
ventricular aneurysm	• reduced ejection fraction • mural thrombi → arterial emboli
pericarditis	• **occurs 1-3 days after MI** • pleuritic pain, non-responsive to nitrates • diffuse ST elevations • self-limited
Dressler's syndrome	• **occurs several weeks after MI** • pericardial and pleural effusions • fever, joint pain • tends to recur

4.9.) <u>HEART VALVES</u>

Signs (●) and symptoms (o) of valvular diseases:

mitral stenosis	<ul><li>diastolic opening snap</li><li>diastolic rumble</li><li>loud S1</li><li>no S3 or S4</li></ul> o dyspnea, orthopnea o atrial fibrillation
mitral regurgitation	<ul><li>holosystolic murmur</li><li>may radiate to axilla</li><li>widely split S2 (early A2)</li></ul> o pulmonary congestion
mitral valve prolapse	<ul><li>midsystolic click followed by murmur</li></ul> o palpitations o atypical chest pain
aortic stenosis	<ul><li>harsh systolic ejection murmur</li><li>may radiate to carotids</li></ul> o angina o exertional syncope
aortic regurgitation	<ul><li>diastolic decrescendo murmur</li><li>"waterhammer pulse"</li></ul>**DeMusset:** head bobbing **Traube:** pistol shot sounds over arteries **Quincke:** pulsatile blushing of nail beds

4.10.) AUSCULTATORY TRICKS

Inspiration: - *increases venous return*
- *increases right-sided murmurs*

	OCM	AS	MR
Valsalva (decreases venous return)	↑	↓	↓
squatting (increases systemic resistance) (increases venous return)	↓	↑	↑
amyl nitrate (decreases arterial pressure) (increases cardiac output)	↑	↑	↓

*OCM: obstructive cardiomyopathy, **AS**: aortic stenosis, **MR** mitral regurgitation*
↑: increases murmur,   ↓: decreases murmur

physiologic split	• P closes after A (inspiratory split)
wide split	• P closes after A (inspiratory > expiratory) ○ pulmonary stenosis ○ mitral regurgitation ○ RBBB
paradoxical split	• A closes after P (expiratory split) ○ aortic stenosis ○ tricuspid regurgitation ○ LBBB
fixed split	• split independent of respiration ○ ASD, VSD

4.11.) <u>PERICARDITIS</u>

Pericarditis pain is aggravated by chest movements (respiration) and can be relieved by sitting up and leaning forward. It must be distinguished from ischemic pain which is not affected by chest movements.

infectious	• **often preceded by "cold"** ○ Coxsackie A and B and ECHO virus ○ tuberculosis ○ AIDS: atypical mycobacteria
metabolic	• **uremia** large effusions tamponade • **myxedema** large effusions rarely tamponade
post MI	• **early** (1-3 days after MI) self-limited, common • **Dressler's** (weeks after MI) uncommon

 ECG shows generalized (i.e. nonspecific) ST elevations.

<u>Signs of Cardiac Tamponade:</u>
- ➤ elevated venous pressure
- ➤ venous pulse: no y-descent
  (impaired cardiac filling)
- ➤ pulsus paradoxus
- ➤ ECG : low voltage, alternans

4.12.) <u>CARDIOMYOPATHY</u>

Cardiomyopathies are diseases of the heart muscle and have many causes:

dilated (congestive)	• **dilated ventricle, normal wall thickness** • **left and right ventricular failure** o alcohol o doxorubicin o infections (usually viral)
hypertrophic	• **ventricular hypertrophy** • **small cavity** • **septum may obstruct outflow** o often genetic
restrictive	• **low ventricular compliance** (restricts diastolic filling) o amyloidosis o sarcoidosis o hemochromatosis

4.13.) HEART FAILURE

LEFT HEART	RIGHT HEART
• dyspnea • orthopnea • wheezes (cardiac asthma) o S3 gallop o S4 gallop o pulsus alternans	• peripheral edema • nocturia o jugular vein distention o hepatomegaly o splenomegaly

4.14.) FUNCTIONAL CLASSES
(New York Heart Association)

Functional severity of heart diseases is commonly divided into 4 classes. This is important to determine patient management:

Class I	no limitation of physical activity
Class II	ordinary physical activity causes symptoms
Class III	less than ordinary physical activity causes symptoms
Class IV	symptoms at rest

4.15.) <u>SHOCK</u>

Shock is defined as any state where perfusion of peripheral tissues is inadequate to sustain life. Usually the patient is hypotensive and oliguric. There are 4 major types of shock with distinct pathophysiology and patient management:

cardiogenic	• **cool, pale skin** • **distended** neck veins ○ myocardial infarction ○ cardiomyopathy ○ arrhythmias
hypovolemic	• **cool, pale skin** • **collapsed** neck veins ○ hemorrhage ○ diabetes ○ Addison's
septic	• **warm, dry skin** • **edema despite hypovolemia** [1] (low peripheral resistance) ○ gram negative infections (endotoxins)
anaphylactic	• **pruritus, urticaria** • **respiratory** distress ○ IgE mediated

[1] *prognosis worsens if septic shock converts to a hypovolemic shock (with high systemic resistance).*

4.16.) PERIPHERAL VASCULAR DISEASES

arteriosclerosis	• atheromas • **large and medium vessels**
thromboangiitis obliterans (Buerger's disease)	• intima proliferation • **medium and small vessels** • common in smokers
arterial embolism	• sudden onset • painful • absent pulse atrial fibrillation → atrial thrombus
Raynaud's phenomenon	• vasospasm of finger arteries • cyanosis followed by hyperemia • precipitated by cold or emotional upset **Causes:** - cryoglobulins - cold agglutinins - connective tissue diseases - neurologic disorders
thrombophlebitis	• inflammation of veins • usually painful
phlebothrombosis [1]	• often asymptomatic • deep vein phlebothrombosis → emboli **Virchow's triad :** (1.) stasis (2.) endothelial injury (3.) hypercoagulability

[1] *Homans' sign: pain in calf upon dorsiflexion of foot.*
Famous, but neither specific nor sensitive for phlebothrombosis...

4.17.) AORTIC ANEURYSMS

A) Aneurysms caused by arteriosclerosis are the most common and dangerous, because they are usually asymptomatic:

ARTERIOSCLEROTIC	DISSECTING
• often asymptomatic	• severe, sudden, tearing pain
• most commonly located in lower abdominal segment	• most commonly begins in ascending segment, then extends distally, proximally or in both directions
• pulsatile abdominal mass	• wide mediastinum on CXR

B) TWO SPECIFIC CAUSES OF ANEURYSM:

MARFAN'S SYNDROME	SYPHILIS
• involves first portion of aorta → aortic valve insufficiency	• ascending aorta • obliteration of vasa vasorum
• media necrosis	
• rupture is common cause of death in Marfan's syndrome	

CORONARY ARTERY DISEASE

➤ Aggressive risk factor modification:
1. stop smoking
2. control blood pressure
3. lower lipids aggressively
4. control blood glucose tightly in diabetic patients
➤ All patients with CAD should receive aspirin unless contraindicated (bleeding)
➤ β-blockers or calcium-antagonists to reduce cardiac work load
➤ Prescribe sublingual nitrates to abort episodes of angina
   (hospitalize if two doses 5 min. apart do not improve angina!)
➤ If refractory to medical therapy: angiography to determine need for bypass

MYOCARDIAL INFARCTION

➤ Establish IV line, give morphine to reduce pain and oxygen
➤ Prompt coronary reperfusion if severe ischemia and within first 12 hours.
   - thrombolysis is relatively contraindicated if bleeding from other sites is likely
      (recent surgery or trauma, oral anticoagulation, cerebrovascular disease etc.)
➤ If ventricular arrhythmias develop → lidocaine
➤ Systemic anticoagulation (IV heparin, followed by warfarin)
➤ β-blockers and aspirin for secondary prophylaxis

CARDIOMYOPATHY

➤ Dilated heart → digitalis, diuretics
➤ Hypertrophic heart → β-blockers
➤ Diuretics (hypovolemia) and glycosides increase obstruction!
➤ Consider septal myotomy in severe cases

HEART FAILURE

➤ Control excess salt and water: sodium restriction plus diuretics
➤ Vasodilators to reduce afterload: ACE inhibitors, Angiotensin-II receptor blockers
➤ Improve cardiac contractility: digitalis
                          (watch for hypokalemia and drug interactions!!!)

ARRHYTHMIAS

- ➤ Drug therapy is often a matter of "trial and error"
  (all anti-arrhythmic drugs have the potential to trigger new arrhythmias!)
- ➤ Pacemaker indications see table 4.4

SUPRAVENTRICULAR TACHYARRHYTHMIAS

- ➤ β-blockers
- ➤ Adenosine

ATRIAL FLUTTER/FIBRILLATION

- ➤ Digoxin, β-blockers, Ca-antagonists
- ➤ Cardioversion if hypotension or heart failure develops

VENTRICULAR FIBRILLATION

- ➤ Cardioversion (300-400 J)
- ➤ Lidocaine
- ➤ Bretylium, amiodarone etc.

WPW

- ➤ Quinidine to prolong AV time

RHEUMATIC FEVER

➢ Penicillin
➢ Continue prophylaxis for 5-10 years after acute episode
➢ Continue prophylaxis indefinitely if risk of infection is high

INFECTIVE ENDOCARDITIS

➢ Obtain blood for culture before empiric antibiotics are given
➢ Start antibiotics based on clinical setting: drug users: *Staph. aureus* (oxacillin), subacute course: *Viridans streptococci* (penicillin G)...
➢ All patients with aortic or mitral valve disease should receive prophylaxis (amoxicillin or clindamycin) if undergoing dental or other procedures.

Mitral Stenosis

➢ May be present for lifetime with few symptoms
➢ Diuretics to reduce pulmonary congestion and edema
➢ Watch for atrial fibrillation → anticoagulation!

MITRAL REGURGITATION

➢ If acute (rupture of papillary muscle): emergency surgery
➢ Vasodilators to reduce systemic vascular resistance
➢ Watch for atrial fibrillation → anticoagulation!

MITRAL VALVE PROLAPSE

➢ Usually benign
➢ Treat chest pain with β-blockers
➢ Antibiotic prophylaxis is not necessary if "click" is the only symptom

AORTIC STENOSIS

➢ Significant risk of sudden death: Avoid strenuous exercise
➢ Valve replacement if patient becomes symptomatic
➢ In children and young adults: consider valve replacement (even if asymptomatic) to decrease risk of sudden death

AORTIC REGURGITATION

➢ Valve replacement is urgent in patients with acute onset
➢ Valve replacement also recommended if chronic with moderate symptoms

PERICARDITIS
- Viral and post MI: NSAIDs. Short course of steroids if pain persists
- Dressler's: NSAIDs. (Avoid steroids!)
- Bacterial: drainage and antibiotics
- Uremia: diuresis, pericardectomy if necessary

TAMPONADE
- If patient stable: get emergency echocardiogram to confirm
- If patient deteriorates rapidly: emergency thoracotomy

HYPERTENSION
- Exclude secondary causes: renal disease, renovascular hypertension, Cushing's disease, aldosteronism etc.
- Diet, exercise
- First line drugs: β-blockers (especially if anginal pain present during exercising) diuretics (especially effective in black patients)
- Other drugs: ACE inhibitors, calcium antagonists, $\alpha 1$-blockers, $\alpha 2$-agonists

ARTERIOSCLEROSIS
- Control risk factors for coronary heart disease

If blood lipids high despite diet and exercise:
- Niacin for all hyperlipidemias except hyperchylomicronemia
- Bile acid resins (cholestyramine) to lower cholesterol
- Fibrates to lower VLDL (triglycerides)

SHOCK
- Rapid volume restoration (blood, colloids, crystalloids)
- Swan-Ganz catheter to determine hemodynamics
- Inotropes: dobutamine and dopamine stimulate cardiac β1-receptors (dopamine also improves renal blood flow!)
- If sepsis: get blood for culture, then give broad-spectrum antibiotics (usually a beta-lactam drug plus an aminoglycoside)

ARTERITIS
➤ Most forms respond well to corticosteroids
➤ Cytotoxic agents if necessary
➤ Temporal arteritis: early therapy to prevent blindness!

AORTIC ANEURYSM
➤ Surgery is indicated if diameter > 5 cm (increased risk of rupture!)

AORTIC DISSECTION
➤ Untreated: about 20% mortality within 24 h.
➤ If type I or II (involves ascending aorta): surgery
➤ If type III (descending aorta only): medical treatment:
  - β-blockers and afterload reduction to stabilize dissection

THROMBOPHLEBITIS
➤ Heat and elevation
➤ Antibiotics if thrombophlebitis is due to indwelling catheter
➤ Low-dose subcutaneous heparin to prevent phlebothrombosis

DEEP VEIN THROMBOSIS
➤ Confirm diagnosis with ultrasound
  (venography is the gold-standard but carries risk of inducing DVT)
➤ Heparin (IV or SC), then warfarin for 3 months
➤ Consider streptokinase for severe ileofemoral phlebothrombosis
➤ If recurrent or anticoagulation is contraindicated: consider vena cava umbrella

RESPIRATORY DISEASES

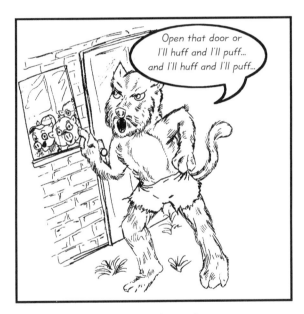

Emphysema in wolves.

5.1.) <u>PULMONARY FUNCTION TESTS</u>

vital capacity	VC = ERV + IC • **decreased in COPD**
residual volume	RV = TLC - VC • **increased in obstructive disease** • normal or decreased in restrictive disease
FVC, FEV$_1$	• most important parameters to monitor in asthma and for pre-operative screening

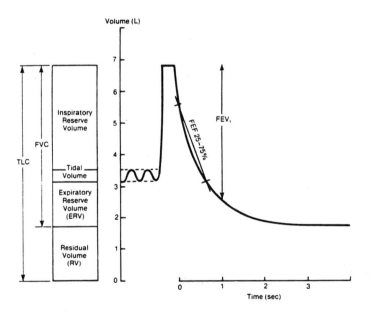

From *The Merck Manual of Diagnosis and Therapy*, 16th edition, p. 609, edited by R. Berkow. Copyright 1992 by Merck & Co., Inc., Rahway, NJ. Used with permission.

5.2.) <u>FLOW VOLUME LOOPS</u>

A) <u>Normal</u>

B) <u>Restrictive</u>

D) <u>Obstructive</u>

C) <u>Upper Airway Obstruction</u>

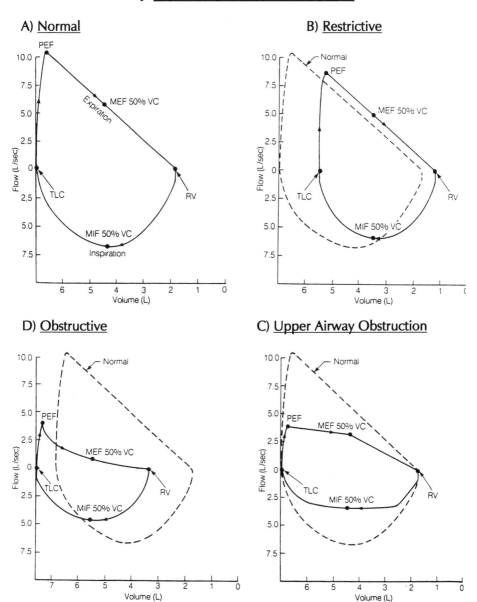

From *The Merck Manual of Diagnosis and Therapy*, 16th edition, pp. 611-612, edited by R. Berkow.
Copyright 1992 by Merck & Co., Inc., Rahway, NJ. Used with permission.

5.3.) <u>RESTRICTIVE LUNG DISEASES</u>

Restrictive lung disease is due to low compliance (stretchability) of the lung tissue.
As a result, lung volumes are low.

pneumoconiosis	<ul><li>**silicosis** (quartz)</li><li>**anthracosis** (coal)</li><li>**asbestosis** (fibrous mineral)</li><li>**berylliosis** (metal)</li></ul>
drug induced pulmonary fibrosis	<ul><li>bleomycin</li><li>alkylating agents</li><li>oxygen therapy</li></ul>
hypersensitivity pneumonitis	<ul><li>**farmer's lung** (actinomyces)</li><li>**cotton worker's lung** (byssinosis)</li><li>**pigeon breeder's lung** (animal protein)</li></ul> <ul><li>isocyanide</li><li>vinyl chloride</li></ul>
Löffler's syndrome	<ul><li>pulmonary infiltrate</li><li>unknown cause</li><li>eosinophilia</li></ul>

Asbestos related diseases : - **asbestosis**: *interstitial fibrosis*
- **mesothelioma**: *long latency, lethal*
- **bronchogenic carcinoma**: *5-100 x risk*

"Honeycomb lung" = *late stage interstitial fibrosis (any cause).*

5.4.) <u>OBSTRUCTIVE LUNG DISEASES - 1</u>

Obstructive lung disease is due to high compliance (stretchability) of the lung tissue caused by chronically high airway resistance. As a result, lung volumes are larger.

emphysema	• loss of elastic recoil • imbalance of proteases and antiproteases • homozygotic deficiency of α1-antitrypsin
chronic bronchitis	• persistent, productive cough • at least 3 months each year • at least for 3 years
"classic" asthma	• episodic wheezing • intermittent cough • triggered by exposure to **specific allergens** • IgE mediated mast cell degranulation
intrinsic asthma	• generalized airway hypersensitivity • triggered by **non-allergenic factors**: irritants, infections, cold, exercise etc.

 Many patients have combined elements of chronic bronchitis, asthma and emphysema (chronic obstructive pulmonary disease).

5.5.) <u>OBSTRUCTIVE LUNG DISEASES - 2</u>

atelectasis	o *airless spaces due to bronchial obstruction, mucus plugs, tumors or foreign bodies* o *often a postoperative complication* **acute:** pain, dyspnea, cyanosis blood pressure drop **chronic:** often asymptomatic
bronchiectasis	o *irreversible dilation of bronchi* • chronic cough, foul sputum • hemoptysis <u>**common causes**</u>: • chronic bronchopulmonary infections • cystic fibrosis • immotile cilia syndrome (Kartagener's)
cystic fibrosis	<u>usual presentation</u>: meconium plug → bowel obstruction pancreatic insufficiency → steatorrhea • predisposition to infections, especially Pseudomonas • elevated sweat chloride • sterility in men • low fertility in women

5.6.) <u>PLEURAL EFFUSIONS</u>

Thoracocentesis and measurement of the pleural fluid protein content gives important diagnostic clues: Exudates indicate inflammatory processes while transudates are due to osmotic imbalances (capillary pressure minus oncotic pressure):

EXUDATE	TRANSUDATE
protein > 3g/dl pleural/serum protein > 0.5	protein < 3g/dl pleural/serum protein < 0.5
• infections • malignancy • pulmonary embolism	• congestive heart failure • nephrotic syndrome • liver failure

5.7.) __TUBERCULOSIS & SARCOIDOSIS__

Sarcoidosis can occasionally be confused with tuberculosis since both diseases have prominent hilar lymph node enlargement. The cause of sarcoidosis is unknown and it affects mostly young adults and African Americans.

TUBERCULOSIS	SARCOIDOSIS
A) <u>PRIMARY</u> • usually asymptomatic • hilar lymphadenopathy • caseating granuloma **Ghon complex:** calcified peripheral nodule plus calcified hilar lymph node	• bilateral hilar lymphadenopathy • non-caseating granulomas **<u>Organ involvement:</u>** • liver • spleen • eyes • skin (erythema nodosum)
B) <u>SECONDARY (reactivation)</u> • multiple foci in apical areas of lung • primary focus often undetectable	
C) <u>GENERALIZED (miliary)</u> • fever, weight loss, fatigue • hematogenous dissemination • pleurisy, pericarditis • meningitis • genitourinary involvement • bone and joint involvement • Pott's disease: tuberculosis of spine	

5.8.) PNEUMONIA: EPIDEMIOLOGY

A) COMMUNITY ACQUIRED:

S. pneumoniae	• causes "classic pneumonia" • most common cause if community acquired • elderly, chronic illness, COPD, cigarettes
Haemophilus	• same epidemiology as *S. pneumoniae*
Legionella	• contaminated aerosols, air coolers etc.
Mycoplasma pneumoniae	• adolescents, young adults • colleges, boarding houses etc.

B) HOSPITAL ACQUIRED:

gram negative bacilli	• more than 50% of cases
Pseudomonas aeruginosa	• faucets, sinks, ventilators, endoscopes
Staphylococcus aureus	• burn units, wound infections
Legionella	• water supply

C) UNUSUAL CAUSES:

anthrax	cattle, swine, horses
coccidioidomycosis	San Joaquin valley (Southeast US)
Hanta virus	rodent droppings
histoplasmosis	bat droppings, (river valleys of Southeast US)
leptospirosis	water contaminated with animal urine
plague	rats, squirrels (Western US)
psittacosis	birds (parrots, pigeons...)
tularemia	hunters (rabbits, foxes...)

5.9.) <u>PNEUMONIA: ENTITIES</u>

BACTERIAL	<u>Bronchopneumonia:</u> • patchy, peribronchial distribution • more common in infants and elderly <u>Lobar pneumonia:</u> • diffuse involvement of entire lobe • more common in middle age adults
- Pneumococci	• sudden onset fever, chills, dyspnea
- Klebsiella	• currant jelly sputum
- Legionella	• diffuse patchy infiltrate on chest x-ray • over 50 strains, wide spectrum of disease severity ranging from acute, self-limited (Pontiac fever) to high mortality disease (Legionnaires')
- Pseudomonas	• common in cystic fibrosis patients
ATYPICAL	<u>Viral or mycoplasma:</u> • interstitial pneumonia • spares intra-alveolar spaces
FUNGAL	*Pneumocystis carinii* • only seen in immunocompromised patients • diffuse bilateral consolidation of lungs • often presents with persistent, dry cough • diagnosis: sputum (silver stain), biopsy

---

<u>What is atypical about "atypical pneumonia"?</u>
(1.) more gradual onset than classic pneumonia
(2.) dry, non productive cough
(3.) minimal signs of pulmonary involvement during physical examination
(4.) prominent chest x-ray ("looks worse than patient")
(5.) prominent extrapulmonary symptoms, myalgia etc.

5.10.) <u>SLEEP APNEA</u>

Sleep apnea has recently been recognized as a major cause of daytime sleepiness and chronic fatigue. Obstructive sleep apnea is much more common than central apnea. Diagnosis is made in the sleep lab, monitoring patients' respiration and blood oxygen content.

OBSTRUCTIVE	CENTRAL
• paradoxical motion of abdomen and rib cage during apneic episode • snoring • obesity, adenoids, macroglossia • Pickwickian syndrome	• sudden cessation of respiratory effort

5.11.) LUNG TUMORS

squamous cell carcinoma (35%)	• central location
adenocarcinoma (35%)	• peripheral location
large cell carcinoma (15%)	• central or peripheral lesion • **tends to cavitate** • poor prognosis
small cell carcinoma (15%)	• usually central location • early involvement of mediastinum • paraneoplastic syndromes (in 10%) • poorest prognosis of all
carcinoid (5%)	• **often curable** by resection • usually endocrinologically silent • not a/w smoking

Stage I	tumor 3 cm or less in diameter
Stage II	tumor > 3 cm - or invades main bronchus - or invades visceral pleura
Stage III	invades chest wall or diaphragm
Stage IV	invades mediastinum - or invades trachea or esophagus - or invades vertebral body - or shows pleural exudate

COMMON COLD
➢ No specific treatment
➢ Nasal decongestants should not be used for more than a few days
(chronic use may cause *rhinitis medicamentosa*)

STREP THROAT
➢ Throat culture if severe or patient has history of rheumatic fever
➢ Group A β-hemolytic streptococci require antibiotics to prevent complications:
- penicillin or erythromycin for 10 days
- if patient had rheumatic fever: prophylaxis for 5-10 years

TONSILLITIS
➢ If recurrent → tonsillectomy
➢ If peritonsillar abscess develops → drain and give parenteral antibiotics

INFLUENZA
➢ Bed rest, analgesics
➢ Amantadine may shorten duration of symptoms
➢ If fever persists or WBC > 12,000 suspect bacterial superinfection: antibiotics

SINUSITIS
➢ **Acute sinusitis:** amoxicillin or trimethoprim-sulfamethoxazole
➢ Adjunctives: nasal decongestants, saline spray
➢ Purulent discharge should be cultured
➢ **Chronic sinusitis:** confirm with coronal CT
➢ Failure to resolve with antibiotics: hospitalization, drainage

EPIGLOTTITIS
➢ Hospitalization required
➢ Get lateral soft-tissue X-ray to assess airway obstruction
➢ Get throat and blood cultures
➢ IV ampicillin or ceftriaxone against *H. influenzae*
➢ Intubation may be necessary (especially for children!)

ASTHMA
- Confirm by spirometry: FEV_1 should improve with bronchodilators
- Advise patient to monitor peak flow at home if moderate to severe disease

- Mild attack: nebulized β-agonists (albuterol)
- Moderate attack: nebulized β-agonists and corticosteroids
- Severe attack: nebulized β-agonists and systemic corticosteroids
- Respiratory acidosis: intubate and ventilate!

BRONCHIOLITIS
- Viral cause is likely in children under 2 years of age
  - Treatment supportive only
- In adults probably due to immune reaction (postinfectious, autoimmune)
  - Steroids may be useful

PNEUMONIA
- Get chest x-ray
- Sputum culture often not very useful
- Empiric therapy based on clinical setting:
  - community acquired (young patient): tetracycline or macrolide
  - community acquired (elderly): amoxicillin or 2nd generation cephalosporin
  - nosocomial: 2nd or 3rd generation cephalosporin, plus macrolide
- Pleural effusion with empyema: tube thoracostomy

BRONCHIECTASIS
- Get sputum smear and culture
- Empirical therapy (amoxicillin, trimethoprim/sulfamethoxazole)
- Bronchoscopy / surgery if massive hemoptysis

TUBERCULOSIS
- Prophylaxis: isoniazid for 6 to 12 months
- Goal of treatment: to prevent development of multi-drug resistance
- **4-drug regimen:** isoniazid + rifampin + pyrazinamide + ethambutol
  (advise patient that orange-red urine due to rifampin is harmless)
- Follow-up sputum cultures monthly

ACUTE RESPIRATORY DISTRESS SYNDROME

➤ Get chest x-ray and arterial blood gases
➤ Mechanical ventilation with PEEP
➤ Monitor pulmonary wedge pressure

ATELECTASIS

➤ Identify cause of bronchial obstruction
➤ X-ray, CT for exact location
➤ Bronchoscopy if tumor or foreign body is suspected

PULMONARY EMBOLISM

➤ Get arterial blood gases and coagulation tests (d-dimer)
➤ Supplemental oxygen

➤ Thrombolytic agents used only for massive embolism with shock
➤ Anticoagulation (IV heparin, then warfarin for 3-6 months) to prevent further embolization
➤ Consider vena cava umbrella if anticoagulation is contraindicated

SOLITARY PULMONARY NODULE

➤ If likely benign (distinct margins, central calcification): watch it
➤ If likely malignant (patient > 35 years, no calcifications): needle aspiration or resection

LUNG CANCER

➤ Small cell carcinoma → radiation plus chemotherapy
➤ Non-small cell carcinoma (early) → lobectomy
➤ Non-small cell carcinoma (late): Unfortunately most patients present with unresectable disease (tumor involving trachea or main stem bronchi, malignant effusions, wide spread metastases...) → radiation plus chemotherapy

➤ Palliative therapy (for bronchial obstruction, bone metastases, superior vena cava syndrome etc.) → radiation

COPD
➢ Stop smoking!
➢ Home oxygen therapy if PaO_2 < 55 mmHg (or saturation <90%)
➢ Acute exacerbations: β-2 agonist (albuterol) or anticholinergic (ipratropium)
➢ Lung transplantation is still experimental and has high mortality

EMPHYSEMA
➢ Bronchodilators (albuterol)
➢ Anticholinergics (ipratropium)

CHRONIC BRONCHITIS
➢ Mobilize secretions (aerosols, chest percussion)
➢ Avoid cough suppressants

SARCOIDOSIS
➢ Rule out other granulomatous diseases (Tb, berylliosis etc.)
➢ Consider biopsy to rule out lymphoma
➢ Corticosteroids for 4-8 weeks if systemic signs are present:
   constitutional symptoms, skin or CNS involvement...
➢ If unresponsive consider cyclophosphamide

ASBESTOSIS
➢ Smoking multiplies risk of asbestosis related disease!
➢ Mortality mainly due to bronchogenic carcinoma
➢ Mesothelioma: surgery, radiation or chemotherapy (usually unsuccessful)

SILICOSIS
➢ Increased risk for tuberculosis: get annual PPD test

GASTROINTESTINAL DISEASES

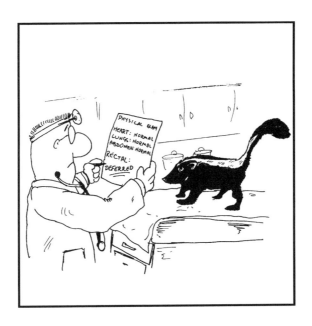

6.1.) <u>GI FUNCTION TESTS</u>

There are several special tests to study functions of the gastrointestinal tract:

fecal fat	• quick test: Sudan III staining of stool smear • quantitative test: total fat in 3-day stool steatorrhea if > 6 g/day

xylose absorption test	• D-xylose is well absorbed but not metabolized
	• give oral D-xylose and measure amount
	  excreted in urine
	• low values indicate malabsorption
	  (e.g. bacterial overgrowth)

xylose breath test	• measure $^{14}CO_2$ in breath after ingestion of radioactive D-xylose • low values indicate malabsorption • more rapid to perform than the absorption test
bentiromide test	• administer synthetic peptide • measure arylamine in urine • indicates activity of pancreatic chymotrypsin
secretin test	• stimulate pancreas with secretin • measure volume and bicarbonate content of pancreatic secretion (duodenal aspirate)
Schilling test	measure radioactivity in 24h urine: **Stage 1** after ingestion of radiolabeled vit. B12 **Stage 2** plus intrinsic factor **Stage 3** plus antibiotics

6.2.) GI BLEEDING

A) THREE KINDS OF BLEEDING:

hematemesis	• rapid bleed: vomiting bright, red blood • slow bleed: "coffee-ground" **source:** proximal to ligament of Treitz
melena	• black, tarry stool **source: upper GI**, or lower GI to right colon
hematochezia	• bright red blood in stool **source: lower GI**, or upper GI if massive

B) CAUSES OF BLEEDING BY LOCATION:

UPPER GI	LOWER GI	UPPER & LOWER GI
• esophageal varices • Mallory-Weiss o gastritis o gastric ulcer o duodenal ulcer	• hemorrhoids • anal fissure o diverticulosis o IBD o intussusception	• neoplasms • angiodysplasias (Osler's disease)

6.3.) <u>DYSPHAGIA</u>

If the patient has trouble swallowing solids AND liquids, it suggests a functional
problem: (1.) esophageal spasm
             (2.) scleroderma
             (3.) achalasia
If the patient has trouble with solids, but not with fluids, an obstruction is likely:
             (1.) peptic strictures
             (2.) cancer

achalasia	• dilated, fluid-filled esophagus • "bird beak" appearance on barium swallow • high resting LES pressure → *biopsy to exclude infiltrating gastric carcinoma!*
scleroderma **(CREST)**	• reflux, peptic strictures • low resting LES pressure
rings and webs	• congenital (Schatzki's rings) • or secondary to reflux disease • asymptomatic, or dysphagia for solids **Plummer-Vinson:** webs + anemia + atrophic glossitis
carcinoma	**Squamous cell carcinoma:** <u>risk factors</u> (1.) alcohol (2.) tobacco (3.) radiation (4.) stasis (achalasia) **Adenocarcinoma:** almost always arises from Barrett's esophagus

6.4.) UPPER ABDOMINAL PAIN

A) ACUTE:

cholecystitis	• cramp-like epigastric pain • **may radiate to tip of right scapula** • Murphy's sign (inspiratory arrest during palpation)
perforated peptic ulcer	• severe epigastric pain • **may radiate to back or shoulders** • peritoneal signs
acute pancreatitis	• severe, boring abdominal pain • **often radiates to back** • peritoneal signs

B) CHRONIC:

reflux esophagitis	• burning substernal pain • **after meals, at night** • may radiate to left arm!
gastric ulcer	• steady, gnawing epigastric pain • **worsened by food**
duodenal ulcer	• steady, gnawing epigastric pain • typically awakens patient around 1:00 am • **relieved by food**

6.5.) <u>LOWER ABDOMINAL PAIN</u>

inflammatory bowel disease	• chronic, cramping pain • diarrhea, blood and pus in stool
intestinal obstruction	• hyperactive bowel sounds
intestinal infarction	• absent bowel sounds • gross or occult blood in stool
appendicitis	• vague periumbilical pain, nausea • later localizes to lower right quadrant • perforation: high fever and leukocytosis
diverticulitis	• steady pain • localized to lower left quadrant • left sided appendicitis"

 Crohn's disease: *- chronic cramping pain*
                                     - fever, anorexia, weight loss

 Ulcerative colitis: *- less abdominal pain*
                                      - more bloody diarrhea

6.6.) <u>STOMACH & DUODENUM</u>

A) <u>GASTRITIS COMES AS THREE DISTINCT DISEASES</u>:

acute gastritis (erosive)	• acute **hemorrhagic lesions** • stress ulcers • aspirin, NSAIDs • alcohol • intensive care patients
chronic gastritis A (non-erosive)	• **autoimmune gastritis** • body and fundus • pernicious anemia due to lack of intrinsic factor from parietal cells
chronic gastritis B (non-erosive)	• **infectious gastritis** • body and antrum • *H. pylori*

B) <u>ULCER DISEASE</u>:

gastric ulcer	• normal or <u>decreased</u> acid production • decreased mucosal resistance • NSAIDs
duodenal ulcer	• <u>increased</u> acid production • *H. pylori*

6.7.) <u>MALDIGESTION</u>

MALDIGESTION	MALABSORPTION
Dysfunction of exocrine pancreas: - chronic pancreatitis - cystic fibrosis **Deficiency of specific enzymes:** - lactase deficiency **Lack of bile salts:** - biliary cirrhosis - resected terminal ileum - bacterial overgrowth	**Dysfunction of small bowel:** - short bowel syndrome - bacterial overgrowth - celiac disease - tropical sprue - Whipple's disease **Dysfunction of specific transporters:** - cystinuria - Hartnup disease

	DIAGNOSTIC CLUES:
celiac disease	• "iron deficiency anemia" that doesn't respond to oral iron **jejunal biopsy:** flat mucosa, broad or absent villi, inflammation
tropical sprue	• diarrhea and megaloblastic anemia several months after travel to tropical country **jejunal biopsy:** may look very similar to celiac disease
Whipple's disease	• polyarthritis • abnormal skin pigmentation, • lymphadenopathy **jejunal biopsy:** PAS positive granules in macrophages

6.8.) <u>PANCREATITIS</u>

ACUTE PANCREATITIS	CHRONIC PANCREATITIS
➤ a/w **alcohol abuse** ➤ a/w **cholelithiasis** ➤ complication of ERCP	➤ a/w **alcohol abuse**
• **elevated serum amylase** • if normal needs to be confirmed by CT	• **serum amylase often normal** • pancreatic calcifications
o 10% mortality rate	o endocrine insufficiency (NIDDM) o exocrine insufficiency (maldigestion)

<u>COMPLICATIONS OF PANCREATITIS:</u>
(1.) fat necrosis
(2.) respiratory distress syndrome
(3.) acute tubular necrosis
(4.) hemorrhage, DIC
(5.) pancreatic abscess
(6.) pancreatic pseudocysts
(7.) pancreas insufficiency

<u>SIGNS OF POOR PROGNOSIS:</u>
(1.) white blood cells > 16,000 / μL
(2.) fall in hematocrit by > 10%
(3.) serum calcium < 8 mg/dl

6.9.) <u>SIGNS OF LIVER DISEASE</u>

	CAUSED BY:
jaundice	• diminished bilirubin secretion
fetor hepaticus	• sulfur compounds produced by intestinal bacteria, not cleared by liver
spider angiomas **palmar erythema** <u>**gynecomastia**</u>	• elevated estrogen levels
ecchymoses	• decreased synthesis of clotting factors
xanthomas	• elevated cholesterol levels
hypoglycemia	• decreased glycogen stores • decreased gluconeogenesis
hypersplenism	• portal hypertension
encephalopathy, asterixis	• portosystemic shunt
hepatorenal syndrome (rapid decline of GFR)	• renal failure of unknown pathogenesis • kidneys are normal! (may be transplanted) • a/w severe ascites • almost always fatal

- *liver cell damage:*   *AST, ALT*
- *bile duct obstruction:*   *alkaline phosphatase*
- *cholestasis:*   *γ-GT*

6.10.) <u>HEPATITIS A</u>

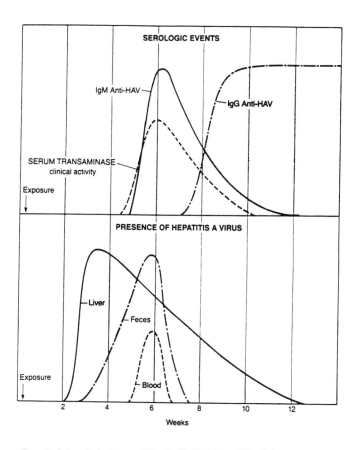

SEROLOGIC EVENTS

IgM Anti-HAV

IgG Anti-HAV

SERUM TRANSAMINASE
clinical activity

Exposure

PRESENCE OF HEPATITIS A VIRUS

Liver

Feces

Exposure

Blood

Weeks

From *Pathology*, 2nd edition, p. 722, edited by E. Rubin and J.L. Farber.
Copyright 1994 by J.B. Lippincott Co., Philadelphia, PA. Used with permission.

 IgG *antibodies: indicates previous exposure*
IgM *antibodies: indicates recent infection*

6.11.) <u>HEPATITIS B</u>

HBsAg ("Australia antigen")	• indicates acute or chronic infection • used for blood bank screening
HBeAg	• indicates high degree of infectivity
anti-HBc	• earliest indicator of acute infection [1]
anti-HBe	• indicates resolution of acute infection
anti-HBs	• indicates immunity (post-infection or post vaccination)

[1] *HBsAg and HBeAg appear earlier but are more difficult and expensive to determine*

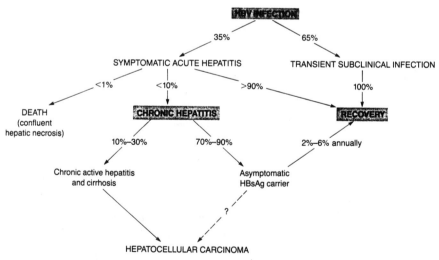

From *Pathology*, 2nd edition, p. 726, edited by E. Rubin and J.L. Farber.
Copyright 1994 by J.B. Lippincott Co., Philadelphia, PA. Used with permission.

6.12.) HEPATITIS B - MARKERS

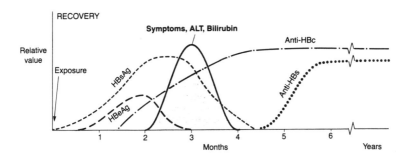

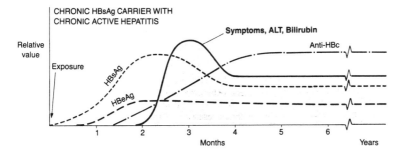

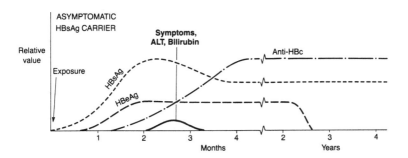

6.13.) <u>DRUG INDUCED LIVER DISEASE</u>

Many drugs and chemicals can cause severe, often irreversible liver damage:

estrogens, chlorpromazine	• reversible cholestasis (→ jaundice, dark urine, pale stools)
ethanol	• fatty liver • cirrhosis (initially micro-, later macronodular)
acetaminophen, carbon tetrachloride	• liver cell necrosis
estrogens	• hepatocellular adenoma (benign)
aflatoxin, hepatitis B and C	• hepatocellular carcinoma
vinyl chloride, arsenic	• angiosarcoma

Chronic liver failure increases systemic concentration of many drugs due to:
- decreased P450 function
- decreased first-pass effect (portocaval shunt)
- hypoalbuminemia

6.14.) GALLBLADDER

Cholesterol is water insoluble and may crystallize in the bile depending on the balance of cholesterol and bile salt micelles. More than 20% of elderly persons in the US carry gall-stones (usually asymptomatic).

gallstones	**75% cholesterol stones** **25% pigment stones** maybe asymptomatic (70%) may cause biliary colic (20%) may cause cholecystitis (10%)
biliary colic	• steady, cramplike (non-colicky!) pain in epigastrium pain <u>subsides over 30-60 min.</u>
cholecystitis	• steady, cramplike pain in epigastrium • Murphy's sign (inspiratory arrest during palpation) pain <u>does not subside spontaneously</u>
cholangitis	**Charcot's triad** (1.) biliary pain (2.) jaundice (3.) fever
sclerosing cholangitis	• autoimmune inflammation of the bile ducts • rare complication of ulcerative colitis

6.15.) <u>DIARRHEA: TYPES</u>

Distinguish diarrhea types by stool frequency, stool volume and water content:

secretory	<ul><li>**large volume watery stools** → danger of dehydration!</li><li>persists with fasting</li></ul><ul><li>cholera</li><li>carcinoid</li><li>VIP secreting tumors</li></ul>
osmotic	<ul><li>**bulky, greasy stools**</li><li>improves with fasting</li></ul><ul><li>lactase deficiency</li><li>pancreatic insufficiency</li><li>short bowel syndrome</li></ul>
inflammatory	<ul><li>**frequent but small stools**</li><li>blood and/or pus</li></ul><ul><li>inflammatory bowel disease</li><li>irradiation</li><li>shigella, amebiasis</li></ul>
dysmotility	<ul><li>**diarrhea alternating with constipation**</li></ul><ul><li>irritable bowel syndrome</li><li>diabetes mellitus</li></ul>

 Diarrhea of any cause may lead to transient lactase deficiency.
(Advice your patients to avoid milk!)

6.16.) <u>DIARRHEA: DIAGNOSTIC CLUES</u>

DIARRHEA PLUS:	SUGGESTS:
right lower quadrant mass	• Crohn's disease
arthritis	• ulcerative colitis • Crohn's • Whipple's
significant weight loss	• cancer • malabsorption • IBD
purpura	• celiac disease
eosinophilia	• parasitic disease
flushing	• carcinoid
lymphadenopathy, immunosuppression	• AIDS (Giardiasis)

 Bismuth subsalicylate may prevent infection with enterotoxin producing E. coli. Great for travelers to exotic countries like Indonesia.

6.17.) <u>INFLAMMATORY BOWEL DISEASE</u>

A favorite on the USMLE - study these differences carefully:

CROHN'S DISEASE	ULCERATIVE COLITIS
o skip lesions (segmental inflammation) o transmural	o continuous inflammatory process o mucosa / submucosa only
• granulomas • strictures and fissures	• crypt abscesses • pseudopolyps
• rectum often spared • ileum often involved	• begins at rectum and progresses • towards ileocecal junction
• **cramping abdominal pain**	• **frequent bloody stools**
	• increased risk for colon carcinoma

COMMON EXTRA-INTESTINAL MANIFESTATIONS:
(1.) arthritis
(2.) sacroiliitis
(3.) sclerosing cholangitis
(4.) iritis, conjunctivitis
(5.) erythema nodosum

6.18.) <u>COLORECTAL CANCER</u>

Colorectal cancer is the third most common cancer (both for incidence and mortality) in men and women. Prognosis depends greatly on stage:

		5 year survival
Duke A	- limited to mucosa	95 %
Duke B	- extends to serosa	65 %
Duke C	- extends to regional lymph nodes	30 %
Duke D	- distant metastases	5%

<u>STEP BY STEP:</u>
Adenomas often progress in a step-wise fashion from hyperplasia to dysplasia to carcinoma. This is due to accumulation of cellular changes:

(1.) point mutation and activation of *K-ras* proto-oncogene
(2.) loss of tumor suppressor genes (chromosomes 5 and 18)
(3.) mutations of p53 tumor suppressor gene

DIARRHEA

➢ Antidiarrheals often unnecessary (opioids: loperamide)
   - may actually prolong *Salmonella* or *Shigella* infection!
➢ If chronic or patient very ill (fever, bloody diarrhea): get stool exam for white blood cells, ova, parasites, stool culture, *Clostridium difficile* toxin and liver function tests.
➢ AIDS patients: often due to *Cryptosporidium*, *Isospora* or CMV

CONSTIPATION

➢ Fiber: 20-30 g/day plus sufficient fluids
➢ Discourage regular use of laxatives
➢ Get drug history (think of anticholinergic side-effects)
➢ Exclude metabolic disorders: hypokalemia, diabetes mellitus, hypothyroidism

OBESITY

➢ Body mass index: weight / height^2 (normal 20-25 kg/m^2)
➢ Attempt long-term eating behavior modification plus exercise
➢ Yo-yo dieting may be a/w increased risk for coronary artery disease
➢ Surgery (gastroplasty, gastric bypass) only for severe obesity (BMI > 40)

ANOREXIA NERVOSA

(Mortality about 5%)
➢ Psychotherapy
➢ Restore normal eating pattern
➢ Hospitalization
➢ Force feeding only in life threatening situations

KWASHIORKOR / MARASMUS

➢ Watch for electrolyte imbalances
➢ Caution: don't refeed too rapidly!

DYSPHAGIA

➢ Barium swallow to distinguish between obstructive and motility disorders
➢ Esophageal manometry if obstructions have been excluded
➢ Endoscopy is study of choice to evaluate persistent heartburn or obstructions

ACHALASIA

➢ Nifedipine to relax esophageal smooth muscle
➢ Pneumatic dilation
➢ Surgical myotomy if pneumatic dilation fails (caveat: reflux!)

REFLUX ESOPHAGITIS

➢ Avoid foods that lower LES pressure: coffee, alcohol, peppermint, fried food
➢ Don't eat prior to bed time, elevate head of bed
➢ Antacids for occasional "heartburn"
➢ Proton pump inhibitors to heal severe erosive esophagitis
➢ H_2 antagonists if long-term therapy is required

ESOPHAGEAL BLEEDING

➢ **Acute:** balloon tube tamponade (Sengstaken)
➢ **To prevent rebleeding:** endoscopic sclerotherapy
➢ β-blockers reduce risk of bleeding
➢ Portosystemic shunts have lower rebleeding rate than sclerotherapy but significant incidence of encephalopathy

ESOPHAGEAL CANCER

➢ If detected early (very rare): en-block resection
➢ Otherwise palliative measures only: radiation, chemotherapy, endoscopically guided laser therapy

ACUTE EROSIVE GASTRITIS

➢ Discontinue NSAIDs or add misoprostol
➢ If bleeding caused by aspirin: consider platelet administration
➢ Sucralfate / H_2 antagonists

CHRONIC GASTRITIS

➢ **Type A:** treat pernicious anemia: monthly, lifelong IM injections of vit. B12
➢ **Type B:** eradicate *H. pylori*: amoxicillin + tetracycline + proton pump inhibitor

PEPTIC ULCER DISEASE

➢ Eradicate *H. pylori*: (see above)
➢ Endoscopic biopsy to exclude adenocarcinoma recommended for all patients!
➢ If refractory: obtain fasting serum gastrin levels to exclude Zollinger-Ellison.
➢ Consider parietal cell vagotomy. Partial gastrectomy with gastro-duodenostomy (Billroth-I) or gastrojejunostomy (Billroth-II) are rarely used nowadays.

STOMACH CANCER

➢ Adenocarcinoma: resect if possible
➢ Lymphoma: resect if limited to stomach, otherwise chemotherapy

APPENDICITIS

➤ Get CBC with white cell differential
➤ Determine hCG to exclude pregnancy if female
➤ If peritoneal signs → surgery

DIVERTICULITIS

➤ Don't perform barium enema during acute attack!
➤ Put patient on a liquid diet
➤ Antibiotics: trimethoprim-sulfamethoxazole plus metronidazole
➤ Consider nasogastric suction and IV antibiotics if severe
➤ If perforated → surgery

PERITONITIS

➤ Abdominal film: air under diaphragm indicates perforation
➤ Empiric IV antibiotics: - 3rd gen. cephalosporin
                                  - ampicillin plus aminoglycoside plus metronidazole
➤ If abscess develops → surgery and drainage

MALABSORPTION

➤ Rule out MALT lymphoma
➤ **Celiac sprue:** gluten-free diet (rice and corn are OK)
➤ **Tropical sprue** (bacterial infection or toxins): sulfonamide or tetracycline
➤ **Whipple's disease** (*Tropheryma whippelii*): tetracycline

IRRITABLE BOWEL SYNDROME

➤ Rule out lactose intolerance
➤ Try high-fiber diet
➤ Anticholinergics or antidiarrheal drugs may be useful
➤ If patient has psychiatric symptoms → try low-dose antidepressant

ULCERATIVE COLITIS

- ➢ Sulfasalazine (5-ASA bound to sulfapyridine) for mild to moderate UC (also reduces relapse rate!)
- ➢ Systemic glucocorticoids for acute attacks (taper carefully!)
- ➢ Opiates and anticholinergics are contraindicated
- ➢ Surgical treatment is curative

CROHN'S DISEASE

- ➢ Sulfasalazine: newer 5-ASA preparations have fewer side effects (does not reduce relapse rate)
- ➢ Systemic glucocorticoids for acute attacks (taper carefully!)
- ➢ 6-mercaptopurine (azathioprine) may allow reduction of steroid dose
- ➢ Avoid surgery if possible. Most patients who have been operated will require more and more additional surgery

TOXIC MEGACOLON

- ➢ NPO and nasogastric suction
- ➢ Broad-spectrum antibiotics
- ➢ IV glucocorticoids
- ➢ If no response within 48h → surgery to prevent perforation

COLON POLYPS

- ➢ If biopsy shows benign hyperplastic polyp → no further workup is needed
- ➢ If biopsy shows adenomatous polyp → perform colonoscopy to identify and remove additional polyps
- ➢ Familial colonic polyposis → screen all family members
  → prophylactic colectomy

COLON CANCER

- ➢ Surgical resection
- ➢ Adjuvant chemotherapy for Duke C and D
- ➢ Follow-up: monitor CEA (compare with pre-operative levels!)

VIRAL HEPATITIS

➢ Bed rest as needed
➢ Avoid alcohol
➢ Nausea or diarrhea → reduce fat intake
➢ Steroids of little or no benefit
➢ Chronic hepatitis → recombinant human interferon α
➢ Infectious patient: isolate if patient with hepatitis A or E has fecal incontinence or patient with hepatitis B is bleeding

CIRRHOSIS

➢ Alcohol abstinence
➢ Reduce dietary protein if encephalopathy develops
➢ Ascites: reduce by 2-3 lb./day (salt restriction, diuretics). Large volume paracentesis (4-5 lb./day) requires albumin supplementation to protect intravascular volume.
➢ Vit. K to correct bleeding tendency (may be ineffective in severe liver failure)
➢ Liver transplantation in suitable patients

LIVER CANCER

➢ Hepatocellular carcinoma: resect solitary nodule. Chemotherapy of little benefit
➢ Liver cell adenoma: May regress following cessation of oral contraceptives. Otherwise resect if possible

CHOLELITHIASIS

➢ No need for surgery in asymptomatic patient (except porcelain gallbladder)
➢ **If symptomatic:** attempt dissolution of <u>small cholesterol</u> stones (ursodeoxycholic acid), otherwise admit patient for laparoscopic cholecystectomy

CHOLECYSTITIS

➢ Place patient on NPO
➢ Broad spectrum antibiotics
➢ Analgesics (avoid morphine → spasm of Oddi's sphincter)
➢ If symptoms don't subside within a few days: definite surgery

ACUTE PANCREATITIS

➢ No food or liquids by mouth
➢ Admit patient to ICU
➢ Nasogastric suction, parenteral nutrition
➢ ERCP and endoscopic sphincterotomy if pancreatitis due to choledocholithiasis
➢ Surgery if pancreatic necrosis develops

CHRONIC PANCREATITIS

➢ Alcohol abstinence

EXOCRINE INSUFFICIENCY:

➢ Low fat diet
➢ Dietary enzyme supplement (lipase, amylase, protease)

ENDOCRINE INSUFFICIENCY:

➢ May require both insulin and glucagon

ACUTE ABDOMEN

➤ Parenteral analgesics or narcotics
➤ Antibiotics only if definite signs of systemic infection are present
➤ Emergency surgery indicated for: perforation (peptic ulcer, bowel), intestinal strangulation, suppurative cholangitis, ruptured aortic aneurysm, mesenteric thrombosis, rupture of spleen, rupture of ectopic pregnancy
➤ Surgery may be delayed or is unnecessary for: biliary colic, acute cholecystitis, splenic infarct, renal infarct, acute pancreatitis, ruptured ovarian follicle cyst

PARALYTIC ILEUS

➤ Restrict oral intake
➤ Nasogastric suction if prolonged

UPPER GI BLEEDING

➤ Evaluate hemodynamic status, stabilize
➤ Nasogastric tube
➤ Endoscopy if bleeding is severe enough to require blood transfusions
➤ Bleeding from esophageal varices: endoscopic sclerotherapy preferred

LOWER GI BLEEDING

➤ Evaluate hemodynamic status, stabilize
➤ Colonoscopy if bleeding is severe or patient > 50 years (neoplasms)
➤ If bleeding continues consider ^{99m}TC red cell scan or mesenteric angiography (often of limited use if bleeding is slow or intermittent)

UROGENITAL DISEASES

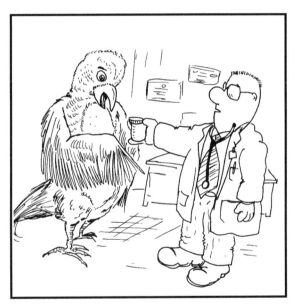

"What's a urine specimen?"

7.1.) <u>URINE</u>

The kidneys produce 1,000-2,000 mL of urine daily and much can be learned from its composition:

pH	**acidic:** - high protein diet
	           - ketoacidosis (diabetes, starvation)
	alkaline: - urinary tract infections
	           - renal tubular acidosis

reducing substances	• glucose, fructose, galactose ○ false positive: Vit. C, salicylates
ketones	• dip sticks detect **acetone** and **acetoacetic acid** but not β-hydroxybutyric acid

casts	**RBC:** acute glomerulonephritis
	        malignant hypertension
	
	WBC: pyelonephritis
	
	hyaline: (a few hyaline casts are normal)
	          low urinary flow
	          hypertension
	
	fatty: nephrotic syndrome
	granular: acute tubular necrosis
	waxy: advanced chronic renal disease

creatinine clearance	• most sensitive indicator of renal function (GFR) (needs to be adjusted for body size in children) • to monitor patients who take nephrotoxic drugs • to determine dosage of drugs when serum level depends critically on renal clearance

7.2.) <u>UROLITHIASIS</u>

Up to 1% of the population develop kidney stones, most of which contain calcium. Advice your patients to drink plenty of fluids to prevent crystals !

calcium	• 75% of cases • precipitates in <u>alkaline</u> urine • **opaque, round, multiple** • hypercalciuria • hyperoxaluria
$Mg - NH_3 - Phosphate$ ("triple stones")	• 20% of cases • precipitates in <u>alkaline</u> urine • **opaque, form staghorn calculi** • following infection by urease positive bacteria (e.g. Proteus)
uric acid	• 5% of cases • precipitates in <u>acidic</u> urine • **radiolucent stones** • gout • leukemia
cystine	• precipitates in <u>acidic</u> urine • **opaque, form staghorn calculi** • hypercystinuria [1]

[1] *congenital defect in dibasic amino acid transporter*

7.3.) <u>AZOTEMIA</u>

Azotemia = nitrogen retention (BUN > 20 mg/dl , creatinine > 1.5 mg/dl)
It may present with oliguria (<400 ml/24h) or normal urine output.

You must distinguish renal and prerenal causes:

	PRERENAL	RENAL
urine osmolality	> 500	< 250
urine Na^+	< 10	> 20
fractional excreted Na^+	< 1	> 1
casts	hyaline	brown, granular

 Fractional excretion of Na^+ is calculated relative to creatinine:

$$FE_{Na} = (U_{Na} / P_{Na}) / (U_{cr} / P_{cr})$$

7.4.) <u>ACUTE RENAL FAILURE</u>

prerenal	low cardiac output <u>Hypovolemia</u>: • hemorrhage • burns • sequestration <u>Systemic vasodilation</u>: • sepsis • anaphylaxis

renal	<u>Acute tubular necrosis</u>:
	• ischemia
	• toxins: - aminoglycosides
	        - iodinated contrast agents,
	        - cadmium
	        - cisplatin
	
	<u>Acute interstitial nephritis</u>:
	• drugs: - NSAIDs
	       - β-lactams
	       - sulfonamides
	
	acute glomerulonephritis
	acute pyelonephritis
	rhabdomyolysis (crash injury)

postrenal	<u>Obstruction</u>: • ureter calculi, tumors • urethra strictures • neurogenic bladder

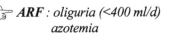

ARF : *oliguria (<400 ml/d)*
     azotemia

ATN : *most but not all cases of ARF due to ATN*
     characteristic dirty brown granular casts

7.5.) CHRONIC RENAL FAILURE

CONSEQUENCES OF RENAL FAILURE	
uremia [1]	• increased BUN, increased creatinine • urine volume may be low or normal • anemia (normocytic, normochromic) • bleeding tendency • peripheral neuropathy • encephalopathy
hypertriglyceridemia	• increased production of triglycerides • cholesterol levels normal • premature atherosclerosis
metabolic acidosis	• urinary pH often normal • diminished NH_3 synthesis (non-titratable acid) limits H^+ excretion • anion gap due to retention of phosphates etc.
osteodystrophy (secondary hyperparathyroidism)	**decreased excretion of phosphate** → hyperphosphatemia, binds calcium **decreased synthesis of 1.25(OH)$_2$D** →decreased intestinal absorption of calcium → hypocalcemia → increased PTH usually more severe in children: • subperiosteal erosions, bone cysts (especially phalanges) • widened osteoid seams (renal rickets)

[1] *The term "uremia" in clinical usage refers to the signs and symptoms of chronic renal failure. Azotemia (increased levels of nitrogenous compounds) is an early sign of uremia.*

most common causes of chronic kidney failure:
(1.) hypertension
(2.) diabetes
(3.) glomerulonephritis

128

7.6.) DRUG USAGE IN RENAL FAILURE

Since many drugs are excreted by the kidneys you must carefully
adjust dosage in patients with renal failure:

AVOID	REDUCE DOSAGE
o IV contrast studies o sulfonylureas o tetracyclines (except doxycycline)	o digoxin o quinidine o aminoglycosides o cimetidine o lithium

7.7.) DRUG INDUCED NEPHROPATHY

penicillin **sulfonamides** **rifampin**	• acute interstitial nephritis
NSAIDs (especially phenacetin)	• chronic interstitial nephritis with nephrotic syndrome
cyclosporin A	• renal vasospasm

7.8.) <u>NEPHRITIC & NEPHROTIC</u>

The clinical presentation of patients with kidney disease can be "nephritic" or "nephrotic":

NEPHRITIC SYNDROME	NEPHROTIC SYNDROME
1. RBC casts **2.** hematuria	**1.** proteinuria **2.** hypoalbuminemia **3.** hyperlipidemia **4.** edema

The relationship between clinical presentation and underlying kidney disease is only approximate. Diagnosis usually requires kidney biopsy!

acute nephritic:
- poststreptococcal
- Goodpasture
- SLE

nephritic/nephrotic:
- membranoproliferative
- SLE
- Henoch-Schönlein

nephrotic:
- minimal change (children)
- membranous (adults)

7.9.) <u>GLOMERULAR DISEASE - 1</u>

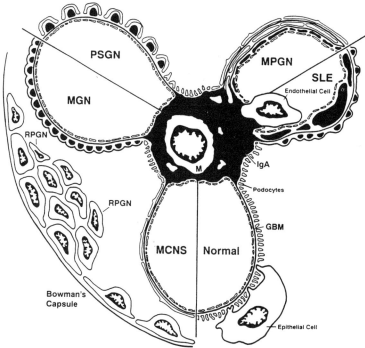

From *Cecil Essentials of Medicine*, 3rd edition, p. 213, edited by T.E. Andreoli et al.
Copyright 1993 by W.B. Saunders Co., Philadelphia, PA. Used with permission.

PSGN: Post-streptococcal **MPGN**: Membrano-proliferative **MGN**: Membranous
RPGN: Rapidly progressive **MCNS**: Minimal change **SLE**: Lupus erythematosus
IgA: IgA deposits in IgA nephropathy

M: Mesangium   **GBM**: glomerular basement membrane

Goodpasture's syndrome (anti-GBM antibodies)	• linear deposits of antibodies ○ pulmonary hemorrhage
Berger's disease (IgA nephropathy)	• IgA mesangial deposits • may follow respiratory infections ○ hematuria ○ mild proteinuria, hematuria

7.10.) GLOMERULAR DISEASE - 2

			PROGNOSIS
minimal change (lipoid nephrosis)	- most common nephrotic syndrome in children - insidious onset	- no immune complexes - **loss of foot processes**	good
membranous	- most common nephrotic syndrome in young adults - insidious onset	- L.M. : thickening of GBM - **subepithelial** deposits of immune complexes - 85% unknown antigen	mixed
membrano-proliferative	- variable presentation	- GBM thickening plus proliferation of mesangium - **subendothelial or intra-membranous** deposits of immune complexes - "tram track" appearance	very poor
focal segmental	- maybe related to minimal change - but proteinuria is nonselective	- segmental sclerosis - usually IgM deposits (**IgA in Berger's**)	poor
diffuse proliferative	- nephritic/nephrotic - **post streptococcal**, SLE	- proliferation of mesangium and epithelium - **subepithelial** deposits	good
rapidly progressive	- aggressive variant of other GN	- **crescents** - oliguria, uremia	very poor

7.11.) <u>SCROTUM & TESTES</u>

A) <u>ACUTE, PAINFUL</u>:

torsion of testes [1]	<ul><li>acute pain and swelling</li><li>**affected testis typically lies higher**</li><li>primarily affects teenagers</li></ul>
epididymo-orchitis	<ul><li>acute pain, nausea, fever</li><li>**pain relief upon elevation of scrotum**</li></ul>

[1] *requires immediate surgery!*

B) <u>INSIDIOUS, PAINLESS</u>:

hydrocele	<ul><li>**transilluminates**</li><li>sometimes a/w testicular tumors!</li></ul>
varicocele	<ul><li>contorted, dilated veins</li><li>feels like a **"bag of worms"**</li><li>may cause infertility</li><li>empties with patient in supine position</li></ul>
testicular cancer	<ul><li>usually painless mass</li><li>sometimes may resemble epididymitis</li><li>**spreads very easily** (avoid vigorous palpation or biopsy!)</li></ul>

7.12.) <u>PROSTATE CANCER</u>

Prostate carcinoma is the most common carcinoma in the male and often localized and curable. It is slow growing and the prognosis depends on stage:

Stage A	• incidental finding (autopsy or biopsy) • non-palpable
Stage B	• palpable tumor • does not extend beyond capsule
Stage C	• extends beyond capsule • no evidence of metastases
Stage D	• pelvic lymph nodes • metastases

 Prostate cancer metastasizes to bones and lower back pain may be the first symptom of advanced disease!

KIDNEY STONES

➢ Colic → immediate analgesia (morphine or meperidine) and hydration
➢ Stones obstructing outflow → surgical removal or lithotripsy
➢ Uric acid stones can be resolved by urine alkalinization, all others cannot be chemically resolved
➢ Screen for electrolyte abnormalities (Ca, phosphate, citrate, oxalate, uric acid)
➢ Double daily fluid intake to prevent recurrence

ACUTE RENAL FAILURE

➢ Determine urinary indices to distinguish prerenal, renal and postrenal disease
➢ Absence of hydronephrosis on renal ultrasound excludes obstruction
➢ Avoid volume depletion: monitor intake/output carefully!
(consider invasive hemodynamic monitoring)
➢ Restrict dietary protein, potassium and phosphate
➢ **Indications for dialysis:** if volume overload, acidosis or hyperkalemia
cannot be controlled

CHRONIC RENAL FAILURE

➢ Restrict protein intake to reduce nitrogenous waste products
➢ Restrict salt, water, potassium and phosphate
➢ Hypertension → treat aggressively
➢ Anemia → recombinant erythropoietin
➢ Start dialysis if creatinine > 10 mg/dl or BUN > 100 mg/dl
➢ Most patients prefer peritoneal dialysis over hemodialysis

PYELONEPHRITIS

➢ Obtain urine and blood cultures
➢ **Mild disease:** oral trimethoprim-sulfamethoxazole or fluoroquinolones
➢ **Severe disease:** IV ampicillin plus aminoglycoside

ACUTE NEPHRITIC SYNDROME
- ➢ Get ASO titer to confirm past infection with group A β-hemolytic streptococci (often diagnosis can be made without renal biopsy)
- ➢ No specific therapy for poststreptococcal GN (steroids don't help)
- ➢ Salt restriction or diuretics only if edema is present

NEPHROTIC SYNDROME
- ➢ Reduce protein intake, unless negative protein balance results in malnutrition
- ➢ Edema → salt restriction and loop diuretics
- ➢ Watch for hypercoagulability due to loss of antithrombin III (may require heparin)
- ➢ Specific treatment (responsiveness to steroids) depends on renal biopsy

RAPIDLY PROGRESSIVE GN
- ➢ Early diagnosis by biopsy is essential
- ➢ Glucocorticoids and cytotoxic drugs (cyclophosphamide)
- ➢ Plasmapheresis to remove anti-basement antibodies from serum

CYSTITIS
- ➢ Trimethoprim-sulfamethoxazole
- ➢ Fluoroquinolones

BLADDER CANCER
- ➢ Carcinoma in situ or early stage → transurethral resection or intravesical chemotherapy
- ➢ Late stage or lymph node involvement → resection plus adjuvant chemotherapy

ERECTILE IMPOTENCE
- Exclude neurological disease, vascular disease, diabetes mellitus
- Nocturnal tumescence to distinguish psychological from organic causes
- Viagra (cGMP phosphodiesterase inhibitor)
- Teach patient how to use a vacuum suction device
- Consider penile prosthesis

URETHRITIS
- Check for other STDs (blood serology for syphilis etc.)
- Ceftriaxone for gonorrheal urethritis
- Add doxycycline for non-gonorrheal urethritis (usually *Chlamydia*)

EPIDIDYMITIS
- Bed rest, scrotal support
- Systemic antibiotics

HYDROCELE
- Avoid aspiration (may cause infertility)
- Examine testes to make sure that the hydrocele isn't due to cancer
- Surgical excision if large and symptomatic

VARICOCELE
- Surgical excision if large and symptomatic (improves fertility)

TORSION OF TESTIS
- Immediate surgery: preventive fixation of <u>both</u> testes

TESTICULAR CANCER
- Get baseline tumor markers (AFP, β-hCG)
- Seminoma: orchiectomy plus radiation
  if lymph nodes involved: add chemotherapy
- Non-seminoma: orchiectomy plus chemotherapy

BENIGN PROSTATE HYPERPLASIA

- ➤ Determine postvoiding residual urine
- ➤ Get PSA to exclude prostate carcinoma

- ➤ Terazosin (α1-blocker)
- ➤ Finasteride (blocks conversion of testosterone to dihydrotestosterone)
- ➤ Transurethral resection

PROSTATE CANCER

if localized:
- ➤ Radical prostatectomy or radiation therapy or observation

for metastatic disease:
- ➤ Androgen deprivation: orchiectomy or antiandrogens or LHRH agonists,
- ➤ Radiate bone metastases to alleviate pain

SEXUALLY TRANSMITTED DISEASES

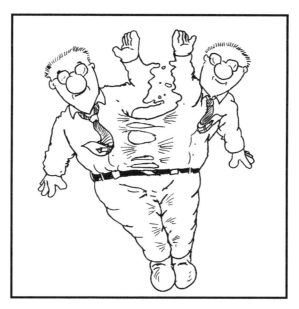

Mitosis – the ultimate safe sex.

8.1.) AIDS

DEFINITION (CDC revised 1993):

HIV positive on ELISA and confirmed by Western blot
plus
- CD4 < 200 cells/mm^3
- or CD4 < 14%
- or opportunistic disease

ACUTE RETROVIRAL SYNDROME:
- fever
- lymphadenopathy
- pharyngitis
- rash
- myalgia
- thrombocytopenia
- leukopenia

CD4 count: - check every 6 months if CD4 > 300
- check every 3 months if CD4 < 300
- start PCP prophylaxis if CD4 < 200

AZT:
- decreases rate of maternal/fetal transmission
- delays progression of HIV infection
- improves survival

Side effects: - nausea, malaise
- muscle weakness
- anemia

8.2.) AIDS: MOST COMMON SYMPTOMS

fever	• opportunistic infections • opportunistic malignancies
skin	• Herpes zoster • Candida • Kaposi sarcoma (mostly in homosexual patients!)
cough	**bacterial pneumonia:** lobar infiltrate **P. carinii:** bilateral interstitial infiltrates or normal chest x-ray **tuberculosis:** focal infiltrates, cavitary lesions or miliary
dyspnea	• exertional dyspnea plus dry cough: think Pneumocystis carinii !
dysphagia	• Candida • Herpes simplex • aphthous ulcers
diarrhea	• parasitic • bacterial (Campylobacter, Salmonella, Shigella)
headache	• bacterial meningitis • neurosyphilis • cryptococcosis • toxoplasmosis ("ring enhancing lesions") if focal signs or altered mental status → get CT (contrast) or MRI if scan normal → get CSF for cryptococcus and acid fast bacteria

 Earliest Symptoms: - generalized lymphadenopathy
                        - oral lesions (thrush, leukoplakia)
                        - reactivation herpes zoster

8.3.) <u>AIDS: OPPORTUNISTIC INFECTIONS</u>
(Prophylaxis)

Pneumocystis carinii	• all patients with CD < 200 cells/mm^3 • prevention of recurrence ➤ *trimethoprim-sulfamethoxazole* ➤ *or dapsone* ➤ *or pentamidine*
tuberculosis	• PPD (Mantoux): positive if > 5mm • anergy control (candida, mumps, tetanus) ➤ *isoniazid for at least 1 year* ➤ *or rifampin for at least 1 year*
Mycobacterium avium	• patients with CD < 200 cells/mm^3 ➤ *rifabutin (development of resistance likely)*
toxoplasmosis	• patients with CD < 200 cells/mm^3 ➤ *trimethoprim-sulfamethoxazole* ➤ *or pyrimethamine*
neurosyphilis	• check VDRL titer once a year • if positive consider lumbar puncture to confirm ➤ *aggressive treatment with penicillin G*

8.4.) AIDS: OPPORTUNISTIC INFECTIONS
(Treatment)

Morbidity of AIDS patients is largely due to opportunistic infections. Despite aggressive treatment, most AIDS patients eventually succumb to these infections:

Herpes simplex or zoster	➢ acyclovir
CMV	➢ ganciclovir
Mycobacterium tuberculosis	<u>Four drug regimen:</u> (1.) isoniazid (2.) rifampin (3.) pyrazinamide (4.) ethambutol
Candida (esophageal)	➢ fluconazole, ketoconazole
Cryptococcus neoformans	➢ fluconazole
Pneumocystis carinii	➢ trimethoprim-sulfamethoxazole (pentamidine if allergic)
Toxoplasma gondii	➢ pyrimethamine-sulfadiazine

8.5.) OTHER SEXUALLY TRANSMITTED DISEASES

	CAUSED BY:	CLINICAL FEATURES:	TREATMENT:
gonorrhea	*Neisseria gonorrhoeae*	purulent urethritis	ceftriaxone
trichomoniasis	*Trichomonas vaginalis*	men: asymptomatic or NGU female: vaginitis	metronidazole
non-gonococcal urethritis (NGU)	*Chlamydia trachomatis* [1]	urethritis, PID	doxycycline
lymphogranuloma venereum	*Chlamydia trachomatis* [2]	ulcer (**painless**) lymphadenopathy	doxycycline
granuloma inguinale	*C. donovani*	multiple ulcerating papules lymph nodes not involved [3]	tetracycline
chancroid	*Haemophilus ducreyi*	soft chancre (**painful**)	ceftriaxone
syphilis (I) **syphilis (II)** **syphilis (III)**	*Treponema pallidum*	hard chancre (**painless**) cond. lata (flat brown papules) gumma	penicillin G
condyloma acuminatum	HPV	"red warts"	cryotherapy
genital herpes	HSV2 or HSV1	recurrent vesicles (**painful**)	acyclovir

[1,2] *different strains*   [3] *induration is of subcutaneous tissue*

Yeast infection (*Candida*) is not sexually transmitted!

INFECTIOUS DISEASES

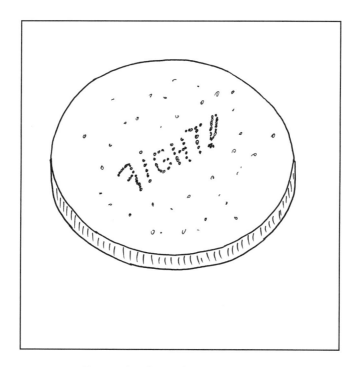

Bacterial Colonial Resistance

9.1.) <u>Key-List</u>

9.2.) <u>DEFENSE MECHANISMS</u>

The human body has a number of defense mechanisms against infectious disease. Breakdown of immunity results in characteristic infections:

	PROTECTS AGAINST:
skin barrier	• staphylococci • streptococci
IgA antibodies	• mucous membrane colonizing flora

cell-mediated immunity	• **bacteria**
	  M. tuberculosis
	  atypical mycobacteria
	• **viruses**
	• **fungi**
	• **protozoa**

neutrophils	• *Staphylococci* • *Candida* • *Aspergillus*
complement	• **encapsulated bacteria** • *Streptococcus pneumoniae* • *Neisseria meningitis* • *Haemophilus influenzae*

<u>DEFECTIVE NEUTROPHIL FUNCTION:</u>
Chronic granulomatous disease - NBT test, absent superoxide production
Chédiak-Higashi - reduced chemotaxis
Myeloperoxidase deficiency - enzyme defect

9.3.) <u>NOSOCOMIAL INFECTIONS</u>

Hospital-acquired infections cause serious morbidity and are often due to *Staphylococci*, *Enterobacteriaceae*, *Klebsiella*, *Proteus* or *Pseudomonas*.

	ARE FACILITATED BY:
urinary tract infections	• duration of catheterization • absence of systemic antibiotics ○ more common in females
lower respiratory tract infections	• aspiration • decreased gag reflex • alkaline stomach pH
surgical wound infections	• duration of procedure • level of contamination • severity of illness **recommended antibiotic prophylaxis:** 2 h before until 24 h after operation
sepsis	<u>primary:</u> • intravenous cannulas <u>secondary:</u> • urinary tract infections • pulmonary infections • cutaneous infections wound infections

9.4.) FEVER PLUS RASH

Some infectious diseases cause skin reactions that make diagnosis "ridiculously simple":

Rocky Mountain spotted fever (Atlantic States, Southeast)	• **maculopapular petechiae** • beginning at wrist and forearm • spreading to trunk, palms, soles
Lyme disease (Northeast, Minnesota, California, Oregon)	• **erythema migrans** (expanding, ring-shaped erythema)
meningococcal sepsis (outbreaks in crowded housing)	• **small petechia** • irregular borders, "smudging" • painful
staphylococcal sepsis	• **pustules**, purulent purpura • nosocomial: indwelling catheters
pseudomonas sepsis	• **hemorrhagic vesicles** • patient appears extremely toxic
candida sepsis	• **discrete, pink, maculopapular lesions** • a/w immunosuppression • a/w broad spectrum antibiotics
infective endocarditis	• **petechiae** • **Osler's nodes, Janeway lesions** • indwelling catheters • intravenous drug abuse
toxic shock syndrome (young female)	• **erythroderma** (sunburn-appearance) • hands and feet • young females

9.5.) DRUGS OF CHOICE

Actinomyces	actinomycosis	penicillin G
Bacillus anthracis	anthrax	penicillin G
Bordetella pertussis	whooping cough	erythromycin
Borrelia Burgdorferi	Lyme disease	tetracycline
Campylobacter	acute inflammatory diarrhea	ciprofloxacin
Candida	vaginal candidiasis	miconazole
	systemic candidiasis	fluconazole
Chlamydia trachomatis	pelvic inflammatory disease	doxycycline
Chlamydia pneumoniae	pneumonia	tetracycline
H. influenza	pneumonia, meningitis	3rd gen. cephalosporin
Helicobacter pylori	gastric ulcer	metronidazole + tetracycline
Klebsiella	pneumonia	3rd gen. cephalosporin
	UTI	quinolones
Legionella	Legionnaire's disease	erythromycin
M. tuberculosis	tuberculosis	isoniazid + rifampin + pyrazinamide + ethambutol
M. leprae	leprosy	dapsone + rifampin
M. pneumoniae	atypical pneumonia	erythromycin
N. gonorrhea	gonorrhea	ceftriaxone
N. meningitis	meningitis	penicillin G
Nocardia	pneumonia	trimethoprim/sulfamethoxazole
Proteus	UTI	quinolones
Rickettsia	spotted fever, end. typhus	tetracycline
Salmonella typhi	typhoid fever	trimethoprim/sulfamethoxazole
Shigella	dysentery	trimethoprim/sulfamethoxazole
Staph. aureus	skin infection	dicloxacillin
	sepsis, osteomyelitis	nafcillin or oxacillin
Strept. pyogenes	pharyngitis, erysipelas	penicillin G or V
Strept. viridans	endocarditis	penicillin + aminoglycoside
Treponema pallidum	syphilis	penicillin G
Trichomonas	trichomoniasis	metronidazole
Tropheryma whippelii	Whipple's disease	trimethoprim/sulfamethoxazole
Vibrio cholerae	cholera	tetracycline (+ fluids!)
Yersinia pestis	plague ("black death")	streptomycin

HEMATOLOGY

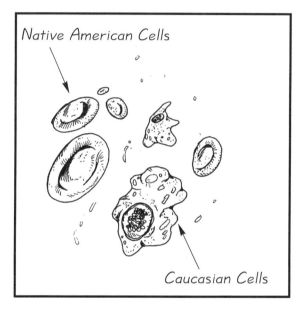

Political Correctness comes to Hematology

10.1.) <u>COAGULATION</u>

bleeding time	• von Willebrand's • thrombocytopenia • DIC, ITP, TTP • aspirin
PTT (activated)	• intrinsic system (factors VIII, IX, X, XI, XII) • **heparin** • **hemophilia A and B**
prothrombin time	• extrinsic system (factor VII) • **warfarin** • **vit. K**
INR = International Normalized Ratio	• to account for variability of thromboplastin preparations • calculated from prothrombin time • benefits patients who travel, clinical trials, and scientific publications
thrombin time	• **heparin** • **DIC**

Prolonged use of a tourniquet before drawing blood sample may falsely increase PTT and PT !

10.2.) BLEEDING DISORDERS

Hemostasis occurs via three mechanisms: (1.) intrinsic and extrinsic coagulation cascade, (2.) platelet aggregation and (3.) vessel contractions.

coagulation defect	• bleeding into **joints, muscle, viscera** ○ affects males > females
platelet defect	• bleeding into **skin and mucous membranes** ○ males and females
vascular defect	• **purpura** ○ gastrointestinal bleeding ○ affects females > males

---

VON WILLEBRAND'S DISEASE:
➢ most common inherited bleeding disorder
➢ autosomal dominant with incomplete penetrance
➢ at least 20 subtypes

➢ prolonged bleeding time and prolonged PTT

10.3.) <u>HEMOPHILIA</u>

Somewhat confusingly, hemophilia does not typically result in prolonged <u>bleeding times</u> as measured clinically:

hemophilia A	• factor VIII deficient • X-linked recessive ○ PT normal • **PTT prolonged** ○ bleeding time normal
hemophilia B	• factor IX deficient • X-linked recessive ○ PT normal • **PTT prolonged** ○ bleeding time normal
von Willebrand's	• vWF : qualitative or quantitative dysfunction • autosomal recessive or dominant ○ PT normal • **PTT prolonged** • **bleeding time prolonged**

10.4.) <u>BLOOD PRODUCTS</u>

<u>RISK OF:</u>

	HEPATITIS	AIDS	THROMBOSIS
plasma	+	+	-
cryoprecipitate	+	+	-
VIII or IX concentrate	-	-	-
prothrombin complex [1]	++	++	++

[1] *rich in factor IX and less expensive than concentrate.*

154

10.5.) HYPERCOAGULABILITY

DIC	consumption of coagulation factors due to intravascular activation of coagulation cascade • PT prolonged • PTT prolonged • thrombocytopenia • decreased fibrinogen • increased fibrin split products secondary to: ○ gram negative sepsis ○ adenocarcinomas ○ crash injury ○ amniotic fluid embolism
antithrombin III	• inhibitor of proteases • blocks thrombin and factor X • potentiates heparin antithrombin III deficiency (e.g. nephrotic syndrome): • thrombosis in young adults • *apparent resistance to heparin!*
thrombomodulin	• receptor for thrombin on endothelial cells • thrombin bound to thrombomodulin activates protein C
protein C	• "the body's natural anticoagulant" • inactivates factor V and VIII • stimulates fibrinolysis • vit. K dependent
protein S	• cofactor required for activation of protein C • vit. K dependent
C or S deficiency	• thrombosis in young adults *oral anticoagulation may result in skin necrosis unless heparin is given first !*

10.6.) RED BLOOD CELLS - 1

A) INDICATORS OF ANEMIA:

hematocrit	• remains normal during <u>acute</u> blood loss! • may be false low if blood obtained with capillary fingerstick ("milking")
hemoglobin	• depends on number of RBCs and hemoglobin content per RBC • each hemoglobin binds 4 molecules O_2

B) RBC INDICES:

MCH		MCH (pg) = **hemoglobin (g/dL) x 10 / RBC ($10^6/\mu$L)**
MCHC		MCHC (g/dl) = **hemoglobin (g/dL) / hematocrit**
	↑	**Hyperchromatic:** • severe dehydration • spherocytosis
	↓	**Hypochromatic:** • overhydration • iron deficiency anemia • thalassemia • sideroblastic anemia
MCV		MCV (fL) = **hematocrit x 1000 / RBC ($10^6/\mu$L)**
	↑	**Macrocytic:** • vit B12 deficiency • folate deficiency
	↓	**Microcytic:** • iron deficiency • thalassemia • sideroblastic anemia

10.7.) <u>RED BLOOD CELLS - 2</u>

reticulocyte count	percent of RBCs
reticulocyte count (corrected for hematocrit)	percent x (patients hematocrit/ normal hematocrit) • indicator of erythropoietic activity • if low in an anemic patient suggests chronic disease, deficiency state or marrow suppression.
sedimentation rate	• nonspecific test • infections, inflammations, neoplasms • increased in anemia!
direct Coombs' test	**test for antibodies on patient's erythrocytes** • hemolytic transfusion reaction (mismatch) • autoimmune hemolytic anemia • erythroblastosis fetalis
indirect Coombs' test	**test for antibodies in patient's serum** • isoimmunization from previous transfusion • Rh sensitization from previous pregnancy
cold agglutinins [1] (antibodies against RBCs)	• mycoplasma pneumonia • mononucleosis • measles, mumps

[1] *don't confuse these with **cryoglobulins** = nonspecific immunoglobulins which reversibly precipitate in the cold (multiple myeloma, Waldenström's, lymphoma).*

157

10.8.) <u>POLYCYTHEMIA</u>

An increase in RBC count and hematocrit. Can be a physiological adaptation to low-oxygen conditions or pathologic:

0. RELATIVE	• **plasma volume reduced** • RBC mass normal
1. <u>PRIMARY</u> **polycythemia vera**	• **arises from a single stem cell** • erythrocytosis (elevated RBC mass) • leukocytosis • thrombocytosis • splenomegaly • may convert to AML *major cause of death: thrombosis*

2. <u>SECONDARY</u>
 	
a) - COPD
    - other lung diseases
    - high altitude
	• **hypoxemia → elevated erythropoietin**

b) - smoker's polycythemia	• elevated carboxyhemoglobin • hypoxemia → elevated erythropoietin

c) - kidney diseases
    - renal cell carcinoma
    - liver cell carcinoma
	• normal blood oxygen saturation
	• elevated erythropoietin

10.9.) <u>MICROCYTIC ANEMIAS</u>

Causes of microcytic anemias can be sorted out by investigating the iron status:

	IRON	TIBC	FERRITIN	ABNORMAL RBCs
chronic disease	↓	↓	↑	
iron deficiency	↓	↑	↓	
thalassemia	∅	∅	∅	target cells [1]
sideroblastic anemia	↑	∅	↑	
microangiopathic anemia	∅	∅	∅	helmet cells [2] schistocytes [2]

[1] *thin RBCs with central dot*
[2] *fragments of disrupted cells*

10.10.) <u>NORMOCYTIC ANEMIAS</u>

hemolysis	• increased reticulocyte count • increased indirect bilirubin *do osmotic fragility test → spherocytosis* *do Coombs' test → immune mediated*
chronic renal failure	• uremia → burr cells [3]

[3] *RBCs with regular membrane spikes or bumps*

10.11.) <u>MACROCYTIC ANEMIAS</u>

RBCs require folic acid and cobalamin (Vit. B12) for proper maturation in the bone marrow.

1.) <u>EXCLUDE APLASTIC ANEMIA:</u>

signs of aplastic anemia

- normochromic RBCs
- hypocellular marrow
- pancytopenia

2.) <u>LOOK FOR SIGNS OF DEFICIENCY:</u>

vit. B12 or folate deficiency

- normochromic RBCs
- hypersegmented neutrophils (band forms)

3.) <u>LOOK FOR CAUSES OF DEFICIENCY:</u>

	folic acid	vit. B12
alcoholics	↓	↓
pregnancy phenytoin strict vegetable avoiders	↓	-
strict vegetarians	-	↓

10.12.) <u>SICKLE CELL ANEMIAS</u>

Due to a single point mutation of the hemoglobin β chain (HbS). The sickle cell trait (heterozygote) is present in about 10% of all African Americans. Homozygotes are anemic. Sickling occurs when PO_2 is low.

SA - sickle cell trait	60% HbA 40% HbS • asymptomatic

SS - sickle cell anemia	90% HbS
	10% HbF
	
	• severe anemia
	• pain crisis
	  (microinfarction of bones, hand or feet)
	• aplastic crisis
	  (triggered by viral infections)
	• auto-splenectomy

SC - disease	50% HbS 50% HbC • moderate anemia • may become severe during pregnancy!

HbC contains a point mutation on the β-chain at the same amino acid position as the HbS mutation.

10.13.) <u>THALASSEMIAS</u>

α- and β-thalassemias are due to decreased production of α and β chains respectively, resulting in unbalanced synthesis and persistence of fetal hemoglobins.

thalassemia minor (heterozygote)	90% HbA 5% HbA$_2$ 5% HbF • mild anemia • may be asymptomatic
thalassemia major (homozygote)	5% HbA$_2$ 95% HbF • severe anemia • requires transfusions • iron overload
α-carrier (deletion of 1 α gene)	• asymptomatic
α-trait (deletion of 2 α genes)	• asymptomatic • microcytic hypochrome RBCs
HbH disease (deletion of 3 α genes)	70% HbA 30% HbH • mild to moderate anemia • microcytic hypochrome RBCs
homozygous α thalassemia (deletion of 4 α genes)	HbH and Hb Bart • hydrops fetalis (stillbirth)

$$\mathbf{HbA_2 = \alpha_2\delta_2 \ , \ HbF = \alpha_2\gamma_2 \ , \ HbH = \beta_4 \ , \ Hb \ Bart = \ \gamma_4}$$

162

10.14.) <u>AUTOIMMUNE HEMOLYTIC ANEMIAS</u>

Caused by antibodies that cross-react with RBC antigens. RBCs covered with antibodies are then removed by phagocytic cells in the spleen (common) or lysed due to complement activation (rare).

WARM TYPE - IgG	COLD TYPE - IgM
• lymphoma, CLL • SLE • viral infections o drugs: penicillin quinidine	• mononucleosis • mycoplasma infection • lymphoma

<u>TWO UNUSUAL BUT INTERESTING DISEASES:</u>

1.) <u>PAROXYSMAL NOCTURNAL HEMOLYTIC DISEASE</u>:
- RBCs, granulocytes and platelets are unusually sensitive to complement.
- Coombs' test negative.
- RBC lysis occurs in hypotonic solution ("sugar water test").

2.) <u>PAROXYSMAL COLD HEMOGLOBINURIA</u>:
- Cold-type IgG against red blood cell P-antigen
  (Donath-Landsteiner antibodies)
- complement mediated RBC lysis occurs after rewarming blood.

10.15.) <u>WHITE BLOOD CELLS</u>

WBC differential is important for diagnosis of many diseases. This is automated by the Coulte
Counter, but if malignancies are suspected, the pathologist needs to see the blood smear!

	INCREASED	DECREASED
neutrophils	bacterial infections • inflammation • exercise, stress • pregnancy • corticosteroids	bone marrow suppression • cytotoxic drugs • chloramphenicol • chlorpromazine • quinine overwhelming infections • disseminated Tb • sepsis
eosinophils	• allergy • parasites	• steroids • stress
lymphocytes	• viral infections • ALL • CLL	• stress • bone marrow suppression • AIDS
platelets	• exercise • splenectomy	• DIC • ITP • TTP

atypical lymphocytes : *infectious mononucleosis*

"Left shift" : *bacterial infection, hemorrhage*
"Right shift" : *megaloblastic anemia, iron deficiency anemia*

10.16.) LEUKEMIAS

Acute leukemias are mostly immature white blood cells (i.e. blasts) while chronic leukemias feature an abundance of mature cells. Morbidity is due to suppression of normal blood cell formation.

ALL (3-7 years)	AML (all ages)	CML (50 years)	CLL (70 years)	Hairy cells (50 years)
fever petechiae ecchymoses CNS infiltrate	fever petechiae ecchymoses lymphadenopathy (splenomegaly)	fever night sweats splenomegaly	insidious few symptoms low Ig levels infections	hepatomegaly splenomegaly TRAP stain!
prognosis : good	good in children	poor	fair	poor
lymphoblasts	Auer rods in myeloblasts a/w irradiation chemotherapy	Philadelphia chr. in myeloid stem cells: t(9;22)	lymphocytes predominate	pancytopenia hairy cells in bone marrow

10.17.) <u>THROMBOCYTOPENIA</u>

< 100,000/μl increased bleeding risk
< 20,000/μl spontaneous bleeding
< 10,000/μl CNS bleeding

THROMBOCYTOPENIA DUE TO:	
megakaryocyte depression	• viral infections • drugs
general bone marrow failure	• myelophthisis • radiation
platelet destruction	• ITP
platelet consumption	• TTP • DIC
platelet sequestration	• splenomegaly

ITP	TTP
• immune mediated destruction of platelets • increased number of bone marrow megakaryocytes <u>in children:</u> • often follows viral infections • resolves spontaneously <u>in adults:</u> • unknown cause • more chronic	1. thrombocytopenia 2. microthrombi → hemolytic anemia (helmet cells) 3. neurological symptoms 4. fever 5. mild azotemia affects mainly young women

Hemolytic uremic syndrome *resembles TTP, except that it affects primarily the kidneys (acute renal failure, no neurological symptoms).*

10.18.) <u>SPLENOMEGALY</u>

Splenomegaly is always secondary to other disease and you must identify the cause:

ENLARGEMENT:	
mild	<ul><li>infections</li><li>right heart failure</li></ul>
moderate	<ul><li>acute leukemias</li><li>lymphomas</li><li>hemolytic anemias</li></ul><ul><li>infectious mononucleosis</li><li>liver cirrhosis / hepatitis</li></ul>
massive	<ul><li>CML</li><li>myelofibrosis</li><li>thalassemia major</li><li>Gaucher's / Niemann-Pick</li></ul>

10.19.) <u>HODGKIN'S DISEASE</u>

The two major types of lymphomas are Hodgkin's disease and non-Hodgkin lymphomas. Patient management and prognosis depends largely on stage:

Stage I	single lymph node
Stage II	two or more lymph nodes on same side of diaphragm
Stage III	lymph nodes on both sides of diaphragm
Stage IV	diffuse involvement of extralymphatic sites

> **A:** Constitutional symptoms absent
> **B:** Constitutional symptoms present

Staging laparoscopy only if anticipated therapeutic consequence. Example: If patient has clinical Stage III or IV, staging operation is unnecessary since treatment is chemotherapy anyway.

Hodgkin's Disease	Non-Hodgkin Lymphomas
• spreads in contiguity • no leukemic component • **Reed-Sternberg cells**	• do not spread in contiguity • often have leukemic component

HEMOPHILIA

➢ Avoid trauma
➢ Never use aspirin
➢ Heat-treated factor VIII (hemophilia A) or IX (hemophilia B) concentrate
  (these are virus-inactivated and safe from HIV)

VON WILLEBRAND'S DISEASE

➢ Minor bleeding → DDAVP (argininevasopressin) increases factor VIII levels
➢ High-purity factor VIII concentrates
  (low-purity cryoprecipitate has risk of hepatitis C and HIV transmission)

DIC

➢ Identify and treat underlying disorder
➢ **Replacement:** fresh frozen plasma, platelets, cryoprecipitate
➢ Heparin is controversial: may be necessary if underlying cause cannot be
  identified, but may induce unacceptable bleeding

TTP

➢ Emergency large-volume plasma exchange
➢ Glucocorticoids
➢ Splenectomy if non-responsive (give Pneumovax before removing spleen!)

ITP

➢ Glucocorticoids
  (decreases affinity of splenic macrophages for antibody coated platelets)
➢ Splenectomy if non-responsive (give Pneumovax before removing spleen!)

HEMOLYTIC-UREMIC SYNDROME

➢ In children almost always self-limited
➢ In adults 80% rate of chronic renal failure if untreated
  (requires large-volume plasmapheresis)

SICKLE CELL ANEMIA

➤ Folic acid supplementation
➤ Transfusions indicated for aplastic or hemolytic crisis
➤ Exchange transfusion for acute vaso-occlusive crisis

THALASSEMIA

α-trait or β-minor:
➤ Usually asymptomatic: no therapy necessary
β-major:
➤ Give folate supplements, but avoid iron!
➤ RBC transfusions to keep Hb > 9 g/dL
➤ Iron chelation: deferoxamine
➤ Consider bone marrow transplantation in young patients if donor available

POLYCYTHEMIA VERA

➤ Regular phlebotomy to reduce hematocrit
➤ Myelosuppression if excessive platelet count (thrombosis risk)
➤ Avoid alkylating agents or ^{32}P: increased risk of acute leukemia
➤ Allopurinol for hyperuricemia

AGRANULOCYTOSIS
➢ Hospitalize
➢ Prompt wide-spectrum antibiotic cover

ACUTE LEUKEMIAS
➢ Young patients: goal is complete cure
➢ Combination chemotherapy
  (Remission induction for ALL is less myelosuppressive than for AML)
➢ Consider bone marrow transplantation
➢ ALL: intrathecal methotrexate to prevent leukemic meningitis

CLL
➢ Most cases are indolent and don't require specific therapy
➢ Chlorambucil or prednisone for progressive fatigue and lymphadenopathy

CML
Palliative:
➢ continuous hydroxyurea to suppress white blood cell count
➢ α-interferon (reduces number of Philadelphia chromosome positive cells)
Curative:
➢ allogenic bone marrow transplantation from HLA-matched siblings.
  (success rate 60-80% if performed early)

HODGKIN'S DISEASE
➤ Stage I or II → radiation
➤ Stage III or IV → aggressive combination chemotherapy

NON-HODGKIN LYMPHOMA
➤ Combination chemotherapy
➤ Regimen and therapeutic intent (palliative vs. curative) depends on disease stage and histology

WALDENSTRÖM'S
➤ Plasmapheresis to reduce blood hyperviscosity
➤ Intermittent chemotherapy (chlorambucil, cyclophosphamide) if necessary

MULTIPLE MYELOMA
Goal of treatment usually palliative:
➤ Combination chemotherapy
➤ Localized radiotherapy for bone pain

Consider allogenic bone marrow transplantation if HLA-matched sibling is available

ENDOCRINE
DISEASES

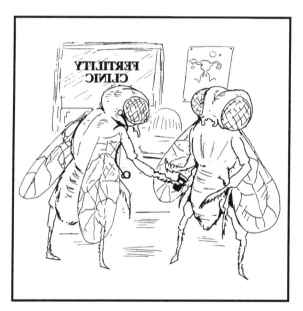

"These pills should help, Mrs. Gordon, but you
might lay up to 20,000 eggs."

11.1.) <u>ANTERIOR PITUITARY</u>
(Hypofunction)

The anterior pituitary controls many other endocrine glands. Hypofunction can affect a single hormone or be generalized (hypopituitarism).

GH ↓	• hypopituitarism in children causes growth retardation
ACTH ↓	similar to **Addison's disease:** • weakness • malaise • nausea, vomiting • <u>but no hyperpigmentation!</u>
TSH ↓	similar to **hypothyroidism:** • depression • apathy
FSH and LH ↓	• early sign of pituitary failure • irregular menstruation • amenorrhea [1]

[1] *in menopause, FSH and LH are increased!*

Sheehan's syndrome:
Generalized hypopituitarism caused by postpartum hemorrhage.

11.2.) <u>ANTERIOR PITUITARY</u>
(Hyperfunction)

Hypersecretion is usually caused by adenomas, very rarely by carcinomas.

GH ↑	<ul><li>**children:** giantism</li><li>**adults:** enlarged jaw, forehead, hands and feet</li><li>reduced glucose tolerance</li></ul>
ACTH ↑	<ul><li>signs of excess glucocorticoids</li><li>signs of excess mineralocorticoids</li></ul> <ul><li><u>high dose</u> dexamethasone suppresses cortisol levels</li></ul>
prolactin ↑	**in women:** <ul><li>galactorrhea</li><li>amenorrhea</li></ul>**in men:** <ul><li>impotence, loss of libido</li><li>galactorrhea</li></ul>

<u>CAUSES OF PROLACTINEMIA</u>:

physiologic	o pregnancy o lactation o nipple stimulation
pathologic	o prolactinomas o craniopharyngiomas o empty sella syndrome
drugs	o phenothiazines o methyldopa o reserpine

Prolactin secretion is under chronic inhibitory control of dopamine.

11.3.) <u>POSTERIOR PITUITARY</u>

The posterior pituitary produces ADH (=vasopressin) and oxytocin.

A) <u>HYPOFUNCTION:</u>

	RESULT OF OVERNIGHT WATER DEPRIVATION
central diabetes insipidus (lack of ADH secretion)	• urine osmolarity increases >50% after injection of vasopressin (ADH)
renal diabetes insipidus (lack of ADH responsiveness)	• urine osmolarity increases little after injection of vasopressin (ADH)
primary polydipsia (psychogenic)	• urine osmolarity >> plasma osmolarity

B) <u>HYPERFUNCTION:</u> Inappropriate Secretion of ADH

signs of SIADH	• hypotonic volume expansion • renal sodium wasting
causes of SIADH	**CNS disease:** trauma, tumors, infections **ectopic malignancies:** lymphomas leukemias bronchial carcinomas **pulmonary disease:** pneumonia, Tb, PEEP ventilation **drugs:** carbamazepine tricyclic antidepressants MAO inhibitors

11.4.) ADRENAL GLAND

Cushing's syndrome	**Signs of excess glucocorticoids:**
	• truncal obesity
	• moon face
	• buffalo hump
	• osteoporosis
	• skin atrophy (striae)
	• virilization, amenorrhea
	
	*(1.) failure of low dose dexamethasone suppression
	    confirms Cushing's syndrome*
	*(2.) high dose suppression test distinguishes between
	    Cushing's disease and adenoma*

Conn's syndrome	**Signs of excess mineralocorticoids:** • sodium retention • hypertension • potassium loss **Causes of secondary hyperaldosteronism:** • congestive heart failure • liver cirrhosis • nephrotic syndrome
Addison's disease	primary corticoadrenal insufficiency deficiency of mineralocorticoids: → sodium loss, hyperkalemia → metabolic acidosis deficiency of glucocorticoids: → anorexia, weight loss, apathy → stress intolerance **high ACTH and MSH:** → characteristic pigmentation of skin folds

Addisonian crisis :
Minor stress or illness may cause fever, shock and
coma due to lack of glucocorticoids.

177

11.5.) GLUCOCORTICOIDS

increased	• Cushing's disease • adrenal adenoma • adrenal carcinoma
decreased	• Addison's disease • Waterhouse-Friderichsen • congenital adrenal hyperplasia

> **Dexamethasone suppression test:**
> should suppress plasma cortisol to < 5 μg/dl

overnight test	**failure to suppress suggests Cushing's syndrome**
	
	false positive: obesity
	              alcoholism
	              depression

low dose test (48h)	**failure to suppress confirms Cushing's syndrome**
high dose test (48h)	*do if low dose fails to suppress cortisol* if cortisol < 5 μg/dl: **Cushing's disease** if cortisol > 5 μg/dl: **adrenal tumor** **or ectopic ACTH**

Cushing's syndrome: *Cortisol excess*
Cushing's disease: *Pituitary ACTH → Cortisol excess*

11.6.) <u>URINE METABOLITES</u>

Metabolites of hormones can be detected in the urine to establish diagnosis of endocrine disorders. Many of these tests have been replaced by direct measurement of hormones in the serum (RIA or ELISA).

17-hydroxycorticosteroids	• Cushing's • adrenogenital syndrome
17-ketosteroids	• androstenedione and DHEA • pituitary, adrenal or testicular tumors
vanillylmandelic acid, metanephrines	• catecholamines: **pheochromocytoma**
5-hydroxyindoleacetic acid	• serotonin metabolite: **carcinoid**

11.7.) THYROID HORMONES

Thyroxin (T4) is converted to the biologically active hormone T3.

T3, T4	increased: hyperthyroidism estrogens, pregnancy decreased: euthyroid sick state hypothyroidism
T3 resin uptake	increased: hyperthyroidism nephrotic syndrome (TBG ↓) steroids, heparin, aspirin, others decreased: hypothyroidism estrogens, pregnancy (TBG↑)
TSH	increased: primary hypothyroidism (Hashimoto's) pituitary adenoma decreased: primary hyperthyroidism (Graves') pituitary insufficiency

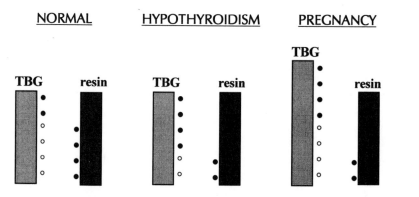

NORMAL   **HYPOTHYROIDISM**   **PREGNANCY**

° T_3
• T_3 (radiolabeled)
number of • on resin = T_3 resin uptake

180

11.8.) <u>THYROID GLAND</u>

Thyroid hormones increase metabolism , O_2 consumption and protein synthesis.

HYPERTHYROIDISM	HYPOTHYROIDISM
• heat intolerance • nervousness • palpitations, atrial fibrillation • weight loss (good appetite!)	• cold intolerance • constipation • coarse hair • myxedema • weight gain (low appetite!)
<u>most common cause:</u> Graves' disease	<u>most common cause:</u> Hashimoto's thyroiditis

Graves' disease	• antibodies to TSH receptors stimulate thyroid • radioactive iodine uptake very high • exophthalmus • <u>pretibial</u> myxedema [1]
congenital hypothyroidism	• cretinism • iodine deficiency or thyroid dysgenesis
acquired hypothyroidism	• Hashimoto's thyroiditis (autoimmune) • patient's treated previously for hyper-thyroidism with [131]I
sick euthyroid syndrome	• T3 and T4 low • TSH normal • no clinical signs of hypothyroidism!

[1] do not confuse with the myxedema of hypothyroidism!

11.9.) <u>GLUCOSE</u>

Long-term complications of diabetes mellitus are due to accelerated arteriosclerosis. Tight monitoring and control of blood sugar levels is most important to delay these complications.

fasting glucose	**blood:** 60 -100 mg/dl **plasma:** 70-110 mg/dl
oral glucose tolerance	• perform if fasting glucose 110-140 mg/ml • pregnancy screening: "Glucola" test.

Oral glucose tolerance is a sensitive test to detect early diabetes mellitus. However, patients with impaired glucose tolerance do not necessarily progress to overt diabetes.

<u>DIABETES MELLITUS:</u>
fasting plasma glucose > 140 mg/ml (two occasions)
- or 1h and 2h values > 200 mg/ml

<u>IMPAIRED GLUCOSE TOLERANCE:</u>
fasting plasma glucose < 140 mg/ml
- and 2h value 140-200 mg/ml
- and at least one intervening value > 200 mg/d

182

11.10.) DIABETES MELLITUS

Type I diabetes (IDDM) is due to immune-mediated destruction of pancreatic β-cells. Type II diabetes (NIDDM) is due to insulin resistance. While most patients with NIDDM can be managed by diet and oral hypoglycemic drugs, some of these patients also require insulin.

	IDDM	NIDDM
onset	juvenile	adult
body weight	normal	obese
ketoacidosis	common	rare
insulin resistance	rare	almost always
identical twin concordance	< 50%	almost 100%
HLA association	DR3, DR4	none
other autoimmune diseases	associated	not associated

insulin RIA	• to diagnose insulinoma or islet cell hyperplasia
insulin, C-peptide	• pro-insulin is cleaved into insulin plus C-peptide • patients with insulinomas have low blood glucose and high insulin and C-peptide levels • if a patient presents with hypoglycemia and the C-peptide is not elevated: suspect factitious disorder!

SHEEHAN'S SYNDROME

Replace hormones that depend on pituitary function:
- Hydrocortisone
- Levothyroxine
- Estrogens
- Induction of ovulation: clomiphene

ACROMEGALY

- Bone growth is irreversible!
- Transphenoidal resection or radiation of pituitary adenoma
- Then follow patient for signs of hypopituitarism...

DIABETES INSIPIDUS

- Central diabetes insipidus → intranasal desmopressin (argininevasopressin)
- Renal diabetes insipidus → thiazides

SIADH

- Furosemide
  (plus hypertonic saline (3%) to prevent sodium loss)
- Correct sodium levels slowly
  (danger of central pontine demyelination if adjusted to fast)

PHEOCHROMOCYTOMA

- Localize with ^{131}I-meta-iodobenzylguanidine scan

Before surgery:
- α-blocker: phenoxybenzamine
- β-blocker: propanolol

CUSHING'S
- Do high dose dexamethasone suppression test if low dose test confirms Cushing's syndrome
- Remove pituitary tumor or ectopic tumor
- If ACTH comes from widespread metastases suppress adrenal cortisol secretion with ketoconazole or metyrapone

ADDISON'S CRISIS
- Obtain plasma sample to determine ACTH
- Perform rapid ACTH stimulation test if feasible
- Administer IV hydrocortisone
- Correct fluid and electrolytes, watch K^+
- Lifelong supplementation with glucocorticoids (e.g. hydrocortisone) and mineralocorticoids (e.g. fludrocortisone)

HYPERTHYROIDISM (GRAVES' DISEASE)
- ^{131}I (risk of hypothyroidism after 10 years: 70%)
- Surgical ablation (risk of hypothyroidism after 10 years: 40%)
- Propylthiouracil is drug of choice during pregnancy

THYROTOXIC CRISIS
- Propylthiouracil
- Propranolol
- Iodide

HYPOTHYROIDISM
- L-thyroxine

THYROID CANCER
- Total thyroidectomy, followed by ^{131}I (except medullary C-cell carcinoma)

HYPERLIPIDEMIA

➢ Rule out secondary causes (hypothyroidism, diabetes, alcohol abuse, β-blockers, corticosteroids, thiazides)
➢ Weight reduction: diet, exercise
➢ Calculate LDL and monitor patient. If diet fails → drug therapy
➢ There is no "ideal" cholesterol. The more risk factors for CAD are present, the more aggressively should cholesterol be lowered
➢ High triglycerides: fibrates and nicotinic acid
➢ High LDL cholesterol: bile acid sequestrants, HMG CoA reductase inhibitors, niacin

IDDM

➢ Provide regular meal times and caloric content
➢ Adjust insulin types and times according to daily glucose profile
➢ Nocturnal hypoglycemia may result in morning hyperglycemia! You should decrease the insulin dose!
➢ Home blood glucose monitoring
➢ Glycosylated hemoglobin (HbA1C) to assess long-term control. Not useful for specific adjustments to insulin therapy

NIDDM

➢ Weight loss is most important
➢ Sulfonylureas
➢ Insulin may become necessary in late stage

MUSCULOSKELETAL DISEASES

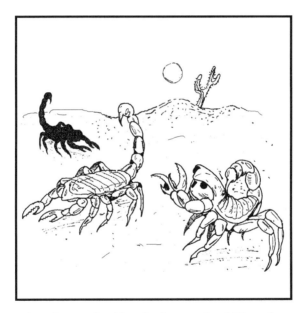

Lumbar spinal lordosis – major killer of
the desert scorpion.

12.1.) <u>AUTOANTIBODIES</u>

ANA	• **sensitive** but not specific for SLE *(for screening!)*
ds-DNA	• **specific** but not sensitive for SLE *(for workup!)* • correlates with disease activity
Sm [1]	• **specific** but not sensitive for SLE
anti-histone	• drug induced SLE

[1] *don't confuse with anti-smooth-muscle antibodies (sclerosing cholangitis)*

anti-centromere	• specific and sensitive for CREST
anti-Scl 70	• specific but not sensitive for systemic sclerosis
anti-SS-A (Ro)	• Sjögren's syndrome
anti-SS-B (La)	• Sjögren's syndrome • less frequent than Ro
c-ANCA	• Wegener's granulomatosis
p-ANCA	• less sensitive and specific than c-ANCA
rheumatoid factor	• auto-antibodies against IgG • sensitive but not specific for rheumatoid arthritis • tends to correlate with disease severity

ANA : *ds-DNA, ss-DNA, histones*
ENA : *(soluble nonhistone proteins): Sm, Ro, La*

PTH acts on bone osteoclasts and mobilizes calcium. Disorders of bone mineralization have a characteristic pattern:

	Ca^{2+}	phosphate	alk. phosphatase	PTH
hypoparathyroidism	↓	↑	O	↓
pseudohypoparathyroidism	↓	↑	O	↑
osteoporosis	O	O	O	O
osteomalacia	↓	↓	↑	↑
Vit. D intoxication	↑	↑	O	↓

12.3.) <u>ARTHRITIS</u>

Please compare rheumatoid arthritis (autoimmune disease) with osteoarthritis (degenerative disease):

RHEUMATOID ARTHRITIS	OSTEOARTHRITIS
• morning stiffness • swelling of 3 or more joints • *wrist, MCP and PIP involved* • subcutaneous nodules • rheumatoid factor • HLA-DR1 and DR4	• progressive pain • relieved by rest • hip joint, knee joint • *DIP and PIP (in women)*
<u>X-ray</u>: • joint erosions • periarticular bone erosions	<u>X-ray</u>: • loss of cartilage • narrowed joint space • subchondral cysts and sclerosis • new bone formation (marginal osteophytes)
characteristic hand deformity **"swan neck":** • metacarpophalangeal subluxation • ulnar deviation of digits • hyperextension of PIP	

<u>SYSTEMIC MANIFESTATIONS OF</u>
<u>RHEUMATOID ARTHRITIS</u>:
(1.) rheumatoid nodules
(2.) uveitis, retinitis
(3.) pleuritis
(4.) pericarditis
(5.) myocarditis
(6.) vasculitis

12.4.) <u>GOUT</u>

Gout is a chronic arthritis caused by deposition of urate crystals, but most patients with elevated uric acid levels do NOT develop gout. Clinically, gout may be difficult to distinguish from pseudogout without looking at the crystals under a polarizing microscope:

GOUT	PSEUDOGOUT
• urate crystals • severe but self limited pain attack	• calcium pyrophosphate crystals • attack resembles gout • chronic phase resembles RA
• first metatarsal joint	• often involves knee joint
• **strongly negative birefringent crystals** (needle shaped, yellow)	• **weakly positive birefringent crystals** (rhomboid, blue)
➢ *aspirin is contraindicated*	

12.5.) <u>SYNOVIAL EFFUSIONS</u>

In patients with acute knee or other joint swelling you need to examine the synovial fluid:

	APPEARANCE	WBC / μl
normal	• colorless to straw-colored	< 200 < 25% PMN
<u>non-inflammatory</u> - osteoarthritis - trauma	• straw-colored	< 2000 30% PMN
<u>inflammatory</u> - SLE - gout - pseudogout - rheumatoid arthritis	• yellow	> 2000 75% PMN
<u>septic</u> - bacterial infections	• yellow and cloudy • gram stain!	> 100.000 > 75% PMN

<u>GONOCOCCAL ARTHRITIS:</u>
➤ always suspect in young adults with acute arthritis
➤ "migratory joint pain"
➤ eventually settles in 1 or 2 joints

12.6.) SPONDYLOARTHROPATHIES

- always involve sacroiliac joint
  (destruction of cartilage, subchondral erosions, pseudo-widening)
- seronegative for rheumatoid factor

ankylosing spondylitis	o more common in young men o gradual onset o a/w HLA-B27 • **always sacroiliitis**
Reiter's syndrome (reactive arthritis)	o more common in men o sudden onset o a/w HLA-B27 • **urethritis** • **arthritis (knees, ankle)** • postdysenteric (*shigella*) • postveneral (*chlamydia*)
psoriatic arthritis	o more common in women o variable onset o occurs in 20% of psoriatic patients o weakly a/w HLA-B27 • nail pitting • sausage toes

12.7.) ADOLESCENT's OSTEOCHONDROSES

Osteochondroses are non-inflammatory, non-infectious abnormalities affecting specific joints:

LEGG-CALVÉ-PERTHES	SCHEUERMANN'S	OSGOOD-SCHLATTER
slipped capital femoral epiphysis (aseptic necrosis)	vertebral osteochondritis	osteochondritis of tibia tubercle
• develops slowly • usually unilateral • more common in obese boys • hip pain referred to thigh or knee	• "round shouldered posture" • persistent low-grade backache • thoracic kyphosis • male > female	• pain and swelling of tubercle • following trauma or exercise • usually unilateral • more common in boys
x-ray: flattening and fragmentation of femoral head	**x-ray:** anterior wedging of vertebrae	**x-ray:** calcified thickening irregular ossification
- bed rest - mobile traction - splints -if untreated predisposes to osteoarthritis	- avoid weightbearing stress - rest on rigid bed - surgical correction in severe cases	- resolves spontaneously - avoid exercise (knee bends) - if persistent: steroids

194

12.8.) LUPUS

Lupus erythematosus is an autoimmune disease affecting mostly young women.

systemic lupus	• **butterfly rash** (spares nasolabial fold) • **discoid rash** • arthritis • serositis • nephrotic syndrome ○ anemia, pancytopenia ○ **antinuclear antibodies** ○ false positive serology for syphilis (anticardiolipin antibodies)
discoid lupus (5-10% → SLE)	<u>Disease limited to skin:</u> • scaly lesions with raised erythematous rim • leaves disfiguring scars • patchy loss of scalp hair (irreversible)
subacute cutaneous lupus	• wide-spread **annular, nonscarring lesions** • photosensitivity • often ANA negative • anti-Ro positive
drug induced lupus	• often mild • **reversible after drug cessation** • ANA may persist for years

---

Common drugs that may induce lupus:
➢ hydralazine
➢ procainamide
➢ isoniazid
➢ chlorpromazine
➢ methyldopa

12.9.) SCLERODERMA

Scleroderma is a multisystem disease with overproduction and accumulation of collagen and other matrix proteins in the skin and organs.

localized scleroderma = morphea	• more common in children • violet, expanding lesions • may be disfiguring if on forehead ("coup de sabre")
limited systemic sclerosis = CREST	**C** alcinosis **R** aynaud's **E** sophageal dysmotility **S** clerodactyly **T** elangiectasia • rarely involves internal organs • fair prognosis • **anti-centromere antibody**
progressive systemic sclerosis	like CREST, but more rapid progression of skin disease and early involvement of internal organs. **Renal crisis:** • malignant hypertension • oliguria **Pulmonary disease:** • interstitial fibrosis o poor prognosis o anti-topoisomerase antibody (Scl-70)

 Raynaud's phenomenon is often the earliest symptom.

12.10.) <u>INFLAMMATORY MYOPATHIES</u>

<u>Characterized by</u>:
➢ slowly progressive, symmetric proximal muscle weakness
➢ elevated muscle enzymes (creatine kinase, aldolase)
➢ biopsy: lymphocytic inflammation

20% are associated with autoimmune diseases: RA, SLE, SS
10% are associated with malignancies: lung, breast, ovary, colon...

DERMATOMYOSITIS	POLYMYOSITIS
• myopathy	• myopathy
• heliotrope rash (purple discoloration of upper eye lids)	o no rash
• facial rash (resembles lupus but involves nasolabial fold)	o no calcinosis
• rash of V-region of neck	
• erythema of knuckles, knees, elbows	
• calcinosis	

 Polymyalgia rheumatica*: - proximal muscle weakness*
                               - serum CPK normal

12.11.) <u>VASCULITIS</u>

These diseases tend to affect very specific blood vessels:

polyarteritis nodosa	• **small and medium vessels** o kidney, heart, GI tract o does not affect lung
giant cell arteritis	• **temporal artery** • **sudden blindness!** o female > male o very high ESR o a/w polymyalgia rheumatica
Wegener's	• **upper respiratory vasculitis** • **lower respiratory vasculitis** o glomerulonephritis
Takayasu	• **aorta / large arteries** • **"pulseless disease"** (upper extremity claudication) o Asian females
Kawasaki	• **coronary artery aneurysms** o mucocutaneous lymph node syndrome o fever, conjunctivitis, maculopapular rash o Japanese children
Henoch Schönlein purpura	• **purpura (buttocks)** o abdominal pain o arthritis o hematuria

OSTEOARTHRITIS
- ➤ Exercise, physical therapy to maintain mobility
- ➤ If knee joints involved: diet and weight loss
- ➤ Selective COX-2 inhibitor: rofecoxib
- ➤ Intra-articular injection of glucocorticoid to reduce acute inflammation

RHEUMATOID ARTHRITIS
anti-inflammatory:
- ➤ Aspirin, other NSAIDs. Consider misoprostol to reduce risk of gastric ulceration
- ➤ Glucocorticoids (intra-articular or systemic)

disease-modifying:
(don't expect beneficial effect until 2-6 months after initiating therapy)
- ➤ Gold, penicillamine, quinine
- ➤ Methotrexate for severe cases
  (used in much lower dosage than for cancer therapy)

GOUT
- ➤ Do not treat asymptomatic hyperuricemia!

- ➤ **Acute attack:** treat acute arthritis first, hyperuricemia later. Sudden reduction of uric acid may precipitate further attacks!
- ➤ NSAIDs except aspirin
- ➤ Colchicine (may cause severe stomach cramps)
- ➤ Intra-articular glucocorticoid

- ➤ **Between attacks:** diet (avoid meat, kidney, liver, alcohol). Avoid aspirin.
- ➤ Probenecid (uricosuric): maintain good urinary output
- ➤ Allopurinol (inhibits xanthine oxidase): for patients with uric acid overproduction

PSEUDOGOUT
- ➤ NSAIDs
- ➤ Colchicine
- ➤ Intra-articular glucocorticoid

ANKYLOSING SPONDYLITIS

➤ Physical therapy. Postural exercises. Breathing exercises
➤ Recommend to sleep in supine position without pillow
➤ NSAIDs. Indomethacin especially effective
➤ If anterior uveitis develops → refer to ophthalmologist

SLE

mild disease:
➤ Benign cases require only supportive care and emotional support
➤ NSAIDs for joint symptoms, antimalarials (hydroxychloroquine) if unresponsive
➤ Topical corticosteroids for skin lesions. Avoid sun exposure (photosensitivity)
severe disease:
➤ Systemic corticosteroids for serious complications: TTP, myocarditis, nephritis..
➤ If resistant to steroids try immunosuppressants (cyclophosphamide, azathioprine...)

DERMATOMYOSITIS

➤ Corticosteroids
  (taper slowly and monitor muscle enzymes)
➤ IV immunoglobulin if unresponsive to steroids

Search for underlying malignancies. These may not become apparent for months after onset of dermatomyositis!

 Thrombosis in a young women: think 1.) oral contraceptives, 2.) SLE (antiphospholipid antibodies). Requires oral anticoagulation!

RICKETS

➢ Vitamin D
➢ If resistant to Vit. D (rare renal tubular defect): give phosphate and Vit. D$_3$

PAGET'S DISEASE (osteitis deformans)

➢ 6-months course of bisphosphates
➢ Salmon calcitonin suppresses osteoclastic activity
  (human calcitonin is more expensive but less allergenic)
➢ Monitor alkaline phosphatase to assess therapeutic response
➢ Watch for renal complications secondary to hypercalciuria!

OSTEOMYELITIS

➢ Aspirate and culture to select antibiotic
➢ Begin with empiric IV antibiotics (*Staph. aureus*),
  followed by oral until 6 weeks after temperature has normalized
➢ Immobilization
➢ Surgical debridement for refractory cases

CARPAL TUNNEL SYNDROME

➢ Relief of pressure on median nerve: hand elevation, splinting of hand and
  forearm, injection of corticosteroids into carpal tunnel
➢ Surgical separation of volar carpal ligament gives lasting relief

DISEASES
OF THE
EYES AND SKIN

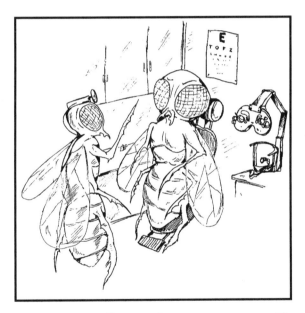

"Now how many fingers do you see, one million
or two million?"

13.1.) <u>RED EYE</u>

Red eye can be a harmless infection or an acute emergency threatening loss of vision. You need to distinguish carefully:

conjunctivitis	• most commonly viral (highly contagious) • eyelids "stuck together" in the morning • mucoid discharge • **usually not painful**
uveitis	• hazy vision • perilimbal injection
subconjunctival hemorrhage	• following increased intrathoracic pressure (coughing, sneezing, Valsalva) • will resolve spontaneously • **painless**
cornea abrasion	• result of minor trauma • "foreign body sensation" • diagnosis: fluorescein dye • **painful** *prevent bacterial superinfection!*
herpes	• conjunctivitis, scarring • dendritic keratitis • **corneal anesthesia**
acute glaucoma	• dilated pupils • **very painful**

13.2.) <u>CONJUNCTIVITIS</u>

<u>THREE MAJOR CAUSES OF CONJUNCTIVITIS:</u>

	ALLERGIC	BACTERIAL	VIRAL
itching	severe	little	little
injection	mild	severe	moderate
discharge	mild	severe	moderate
preauricular LN	negative	negative	enlarged
associated with	hay fever		sore throat
treatment	*steroids antihistamines*	*topical antibiotics*	*preventive*

 In elderly people conjunctivitis is often due to dryness caused by inadequate tearing and can be treated with "artificial tears".

13.3.) <u>GLAUCOMA</u>

Acute closed angle glaucoma is a medical emergency! Loss of vision due to open angle glaucoma can be largely prevented by regular eye check-ups (measurement of ocular pressure).

open angle	<ul><li>**asymptomatic until late stage**</li><li>gradual loss of peripheral vision ("tunnel vision")</li><li>some have elevated ocular pressures</li><li>some have normal ocular pressures</li></ul>
closed angle	<ul><li>**rapid onset**</li><li>**severe pain**</li><li>blurred vision</li><li>reddened eye</li><li>dilated, non-reactive pupils</li></ul><ul><li>○ due to blockage of aqueous drainage</li><li>○ may be precipitated by pupil dilation (atropine)</li></ul>

13.4.) RETINA

hypertensive retinopathy	• "copper wire arterioles" • "cotton wool spots" • vein indentations at a-v crossings • edematous papilla
diabetic retinopathy	• microaneurysms • new vessel formation • "cotton wool spots"
senile macular degeneration	• **slow painless loss of central visual acuity** • pigment disturbances • exudative mounds • scar formation
retinal detachment	• **painless** • flashes of light, blurred vision • retinal irregularities, breaks and detachments
optic neuritis	• **painful sudden loss of vision** • optic disc swollen • flame shaped hemorrhages
central retinal artery occlusion	• **painless sudden loss of vision** • optic disc pale • cherry red fovea • vessels appear bloodless
central retinal vein occlusion	• **painless gradual loss of vision** • a/w diabetes, glaucoma, high blood viscosity • tortuous, distended veins • numerous retinal hemorrhages

13.5.) DERMATITIS

acute contact dermatitis	*"a rash that itches"* Irritants: • soap • detergents Allergens: • poison ivy • metals • drugs
atopic dermatitis	*"an itch that rashes"* • a/w asthma, hay fever • worsened by stress, premenstrual
seborrheic dermatitis	• scaly, oily patches • slight erythema at base o scalp o eye brows o retroauricular o presternal
stasis dermatitis	• venous stasis, thrombophlebitis • deposition of hemosiderin • ulceration o typically just above medial malleolus
lichen simplex	• results from chronic scratching and rubbing • large, circumscribed scaling patches • skin thickening

13.6.) <u>SKIN TUMORS</u>

seborrheic keratosis ("senile warts")	• benign epidermal tumors • very common in the elderly • multiple occurrence • usually pigmented, scaly
actinic keratosis	• scaly red patches on sun exposed areas • may develop into squamous cell carcinoma (risk about 1%)
squamous cell carcinoma	• ulcerated erosion or nodule
keratoacanthoma	• subtype of squamous cell carcinoma • berry like nodule • grows very rapidly
basal cell carcinoma	<u>Nodular type</u>: • translucent, pearly, white appearance • raised borders • may be ulcerated • bleeds easily <u>Superficial type</u>: • scaly red patch • well demarcated
melanoma	<u>Compared to simple nevus</u>: **A** symmetrical **B** orders irregular, notched **C** olor: various shades of brown **D** iameter increasing **Metastases: skin, brain, fetus**

 Avoid UV-B. Use sunscreen, especially at young age!

13.7.) <u>VASCULAR TUMORS</u>

Vascular tumors are usually benign and of cosmetic concern only. Sturge-Weber is more serious because of its location:

capillary hemangiomas	• malformation of capillaries **nevus flammeus** • spontaneous regression **"port-wine stain"** • form of nevus flammeus that does not regress **"strawberry" hemangiomas** • rapid growth for 3-6 months • usually complete regression in one year
cavernous hemangiomas	• malformation of larger blood vessels • **superficial:** bright, red color • **deep ones:** bluish color • do not regress spontaneously
Sturge-Weber	• follows trigeminal distribution • cutaneous hemangiomas • leptomeningeal hemangiomas • possible degeneration of cerebral cortex (→ seizures, hemiplegia)

13.8.) <u>OTHER SKIN DISEASES</u>

pemphigus	• vesicles on mucosa • autoantibodies against intercellular junctions of keratinocytes *TX: hospitalization, systemic corticosteroids* *immunosuppression, plasmapheresis*
pemphigoid	• like pemphigus, but larger bullae on abdomen, groin • more common in the elderly • not life-threatening *TX: systemic corticosteroids*
impetigo	• honey colored crust, superficial skin infection • *Staph. aureus* (or β-hemolytic streptococci) *TX: β-lactamase resistant penicillin or cephalosporin*
pityriasis	• egg-shaped, rose colored herald patch on trunk • followed by smaller lesions spreading along flexural lines *TX: none, resolves spontaneously*
rosacea	• telangiectasia, erythema, papules and pustules (face and nose) • looks like acne, but no comedones • may result in nose tissue hypertrophy (rhinophyma) *TX: metronidazole, wide spectrum antibiotics* *corticosteroids are contraindicated!*
scabies	• parasitic skin infection (mites) • intense itch, burrows • spares face *TX: Lindane or Elimite cream.* *Mites don't survive off body*

CHALAZION / STYE
- **Chalazion** = internal hordeolum (Meibomian gland)
- **Stye** = external hordeolum (glands of Zeiss or Moll)
- Treatment is the same: warm compresses and topical antibiotics

OPEN ANGLE GLAUCOMA
(Non-urgent)
- Control intraocular pressure (IOP): medical or laser
- Regular assessment of IOP and visual fields

CLOSED ANGLE GLAUCOMA
(Ophthalmic emergency!)
- Induce miosis: pilocarpine or carbachol
- Reduce aqueous production: β-blocker or carbonic anhydrase inhibitor
- Urgent referral to ophthalmologist: laser iridectomy (both eyes!)

CATARACT
- Chronic pupillary dilation may help
- Lens extraction (age is no contraindication)
- Corticosteroids for uveitis

DIABETIC RETINOPATHY
- Annual ophthalmoscopic exam
- Sugar control retards, but does not reverse retinopathy
- Photocoagulation to diminish neovascularization

RETINA DETACHMENT
- Ophthalmic emergency, even if small (entire retina may detach!)
- Hospitalize patient, keep head elevated, eye patches
- Urgent surgical reattachment

ACNE

- ➤ Topical benzyl peroxide
- ➤ Retinoic acid cream or antibiotics
- ➤ Oral isotretinoin for severe pustular acne

CONTACT DERMATITIS

- ➤ Remove offending agent
  (antihistamines or desensitization are ineffective)
- ➤ Topical steroids are effective in dry phase
  (ineffective in blistering phase, consider systemic if severe)

SEBORRHEIC DERMATITIS

- ➤ Daily zinc, selenium, sulfur, tar shampoos
- ➤ Ketoconazole cream
- ➤ Topical hydrocortisone
  (avoid fluorinated corticosteroids → skin atrophy)

PSORIASIS

- ➤ Lubrication, keratolysis
- ➤ Topical corticosteroids (avoid systemic steroids)
- ➤ PUVA: oral psoralen and ultraviolet A radiation
- ➤ For severe disabling cases consider methotrexate

CANDIDIASIS

> Oral (thrush): nystatin suspension
> Cutaneous: nystatin powder
> Systemic: fluconazole or amphotericin B

SECONDARY SYPHILIS

> Penicillin. Watch out for Herxheimer reaction [1]
> Tetracycline or erythromycin if allergic to penicillin

STASIS ULCER

> Leg elevation, compression bandage to reduce edema
> Skin care: - lubricants
>   - zinc oxide paste for ulcer
> Consider surgical removal of varicose veins

[1] *fever, headache and malaise 6-12h after treatment*

ACTINIC KERATOSIS

> Cryotherapy (liquid nitrogen) if only few lesions present
> If proliferative (risk of squamous cell carcinoma): wide excision

MALIGNANT MELANOMA

> Prognosis depends on depth of invasion
> Excisional biopsy (1-2 cm margins)
> If thin melanomas are completely excised patient can be considered "cured" but has a 10-fold higher risk of developing another melanoma
> If metastatic: radiotherapy and chemotherapy only of palliative value

KAPOSI SARCOMA

> Cryotherapy or electrocoagulation for superficial lesions

Careful: Antineoplastic drugs in AIDS patients will further weaken immune system.

MALIGNANCIES

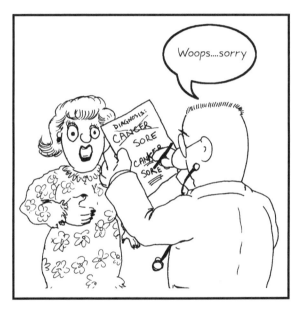

The hazards of poor spelling.

14.1.) <u>Key-List</u>

14.2.) <u>CANCER STATISTICS (USA)</u>

The most common cancer is basal cell carcinoma of the skin. Because of its low metastatic potential (<0.01%) it is not considered on "cancer statistics".

A.) <u>Incidence</u>

> *number of <u>new</u> people that develop disease in one year per 100,000 population*

MALE	FEMALE
1. prostate (41%)	1. breast (31%)
2. lung (13%)	2. lung (13%)
3. colorectal (9%)	3. colorectal (11%)

B.) <u>Mortality</u>

> *number of people who die of disease in one year per 100,000 population*

MALE	FEMALE
1. lung (32%)	1. lung (25%)
2. prostate (14%)	2. breast (17%)
3. colorectal (9%)	3. colon (10%)

C.) <u>Prevalence</u>

> *number of people who have disease at a given date (or time interval) per 100,000 population*

> Prevalence depends on both incidence and duration of disease!

14.3.) <u>TUMOR MARKERS</u>

occult blood	• positive if > 50 ml bleed • false negative: dietary vit. C • false positive: dietary meat, iron
PSA	• **prostate carcinoma** o more sensitive than acid phosphatase
CEA	• **adenocarcinomas (colon, pancreas, lung)** o non-neoplastic liver disease o Crohn's disease, ulcerative colitis
CA-125	• **ovarian cancer**
alpha-FP	• **hepatoma** o testicular tumor o neural tube defects o fetal death
alkaline phosphatase	• **obstructive biliary disease** • **bone metastases** o Paget's disease
acid phosphatase	o (benign prostatic hypertrophy) • **prostate carcinoma**

 None of these markers should be used for screening of otherwise asymptomatic patients (except possibly PSA).

14.4.) <u>PARANEOPLASTIC SYNDROMES</u>

Metabolic or neurological conditions not due to the local tumor growth.
Sometimes, these can be the first sign of malignancy!

DIC	• leukemias, lymphomas • adenocarcinomas
hypercalcemia	• squamous cell carcinoma (lung)
hypoglycemia	• insulinoma • mesenchymal tumors
thrombosis (Trousseau's syndrome)	• mucinous adenocarcinomas • myeloproliferative disorders
dermatomyositis	• breast and lung cancer
acanthosis nigricans	• stomach cancer
myasthenia (Eaton-Lambert syndrome)	• small cell carcinoma (lung)

14.5.) <u>PARAENDOCRINE SYNDROMES</u>

Some tumors secrete hormones or hormone-like peptides mimicking endocrine diseases:

SIADH	• small cell carcinoma (lung)
Cushing's	• small cell carcinoma (lung)
flushing	• carcinoid
gynecomastia	• germ cell tumors • large cell carcinoma (lung)

<u>GYNECOLOGY</u>

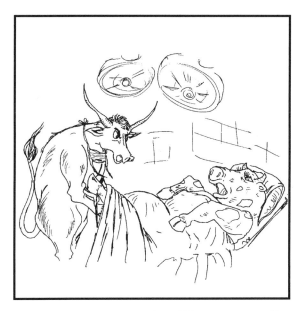

"Relax, Mrs. Benson. Don't have a cow."

15.1.) <u>SEX HORMONES</u>

hCG	**pregnancy** urine: positive 3-4 weeks postconception serum RIA: positive on day 8 postconception • hydatidiform mole • choriocarcinoma
FSH	**acts on granulosa cells:** → stimulates formation of LH receptors → stimulates aromatization (testosterone → estradiol)
LH	**acts on theca cells:** → stimulates synthesis of testosterone **acts on granulosa cells:** → transformation to corpus luteum
estrone	• principal estrogen of **menopause** • from peripheral conversion of androstenedione
estradiol	• **more potent** than estrone or estriol • ovarian, testicular and adrenal tumors
estriol	• mainly produced in **placenta**, but also requires **fetus** • used to monitor fetal well-being in high risk pregnancies

Remember these characteristic changes in hormone levels:

	FSH	LH
prepuberty	↓	↓
Stein-Leventhal	↓	↑
menopause	↑	↑

15.2.) <u>TANNER STAGES</u>

Puberty develops in the following predictable sequence:
breast budding → pubic hair → growth spurt → axillary hair → menarche

	MALE	FEMALE
1	• prepubertal • no pubic hair	• no breasts • no pubic hair
2	• testicles enlarge • scrotum reddens • some downy hair	• **breasts bud** • some downy hair
3	• some coarse, curly hair	• **enlargement of areolae** • breasts and areolae same level • some coarse, curly hair
4	• adult type hair (mons only)	• **areolae project above breasts** • adult type hair (mons only)
5	• hair spreads to medial thigh	• full breasts • hair spreads to medial thigh

 Menarche occurs at Tanner stage 3

 <u>Peak of growth spurt</u>:
Female: Tanner 2 (age 12)
Male: Tanner 4 (age 14)

15.3.) <u>MENSTRUATION</u>

Menarche occurs in average at age 13. Earlier onset is associated with living in cities and obesity. Menstrual cycles are irregular during the first few years due to anovulation.

amenorrhea	<u>primary</u>:
	• absence of menses by **age 16**
	  if secondary sexual characteristics present
	• absence of menses by **age 14**
	  if secondary sexual characteristics absent
	
	<u>secondary</u>:
	• absence of menses more than 3 cycles

polymenorrhea	• intervals < 22 days
oligomenorrhea	• intervals > 40 days
hypomenorrhea	• regular bleeding, decreased amount
metrorrhagia	• irregular bleeding, normal amount
menorrhagia	• prolonged and excessive bleeding
DUB (dysfunctional uterine bleeding)	• excessive uterine bleeding • usually **anovulatory** (= estrogen breakthrough bleeding)

 Average is 30-50 ml blood over 4-5 days.

15.4.) PRIMARY AMENORRHEA

Amenorrhea indicates a failure of the hypothalamic-pituitary-gonadal axis. It is primary if menarche has not occurred by age 16 years. Examine patient for secondary sexual characteristics, signs of virilization and genetic abnormalities:

CAUSES OF PRIMARY AMENORRHEA:

Turner [1]	XO
testicular feminization	XY, testosterone receptor defect [2]
Müllerian dysgenesis	• absence of tubes, uterus, cervix, upper vagina
Stein-Leventhal (polycystic ovaries)	• infertility, hirsutism, endometrial hyperplasia • high LH, androgens, estrogens • low or normal FSH
Kallman syndrome	• anosmia • lack of GnRH
imperforate hymen	• monthly abdominal pain but no menses

[1] most common cause of primary amenorrhea

[2] testicles should be removed after full feminization is achieved !

225

15.5.) SECONDARY AMENORRHEA

No menses for 3 or more months in women who menstruated previously. You must rule out pregnancy (most common cause of secondary amenorrhea). Chronic anovulation is the second most common cause: get progesterone challenge test.

stress, exercise	• leads to reduced GnRH levels
anorexia nervosa	• leads to reduced GnRH levels
post-pill	• should last not longer than 6 months !
drugs	➢ antipsychotics ➢ tricyclic antidepressants ➢ benzodiazepines ➢ reserpine
Sheehan's syndrome	• low FSH and LH
pituitary neoplasms	• increased prolactin

PROGESTERONE CHALLENGE TEST:

positive if bleeding occurs:
→ patient is anovulatory
   (no corpus luteum, no secretory transformation of endometrium)

negative if no bleeding within 2 weeks:
→ determine FSH levels
→ get CT scan of sella turcica

15.6.) <u>MENOPAUSE</u>

- premature if age < 40 years

- follicles become less sensitive to gonadotropins
- **estrogen decreases**
- **LH and FSH increase** (up to 20 fold)

- vaginal bleeding due to unopposed estrogen normal for up to 12 months
- if vaginal bleeding continues > 12 months: rule out endometrial pathology

<u>ESTROGEN REPLACEMENT THERAPY:</u>

ADVANTAGES	DISADVANTAGES
Relief of menopausal symptoms • eliminates hot flashes • prevents atrophic vagina	**Slightly increased cancer risk** • endometrial carcinoma: 4-8 fold • breast cancer: (controversial)
Prevention of cardiovascular disease • decreases LDL • increases HDL	- increased risk of thrombosis - may cause cholestasis
Prevention of osteoporosis • most effective if started early	

15.7.) <u>CONTRACEPTION</u>

No method but abstinence is 100% safe!!!

	ESTIMATED PREGNANCY RATE (during first year of "typical" use)
no method	85%
withdrawal method	25%
rhythm method	20%
diaphragm	20%
condom	15%
oral contraceptives	6%
IUD	4%
depot-progesterones (Norplant)	< 0.5%

 Signs of ovulation *: - basal temperature increase by $0.5\text{-}1^{o}F$*
- cervical mucus thin, watery, stretchy
("Spinnbarkeit")

<u>**Contraindications for oral contraceptives:**</u>
(1.) pregnancy
(2.) impaired liver function
(3.) thrombophlebitis
(4.) breast cancer, endometrial cancer

15.8.) <u>INFERTILITY</u>

Infertility affects up to 20% of couples in the US and should be investigated if conception fails after 1 year of unprotected intercourse.

pelvic abnormalities	• congenital abnormalities • salpingitis (gonorrhea, chlamydia) • endometriosis
anovulation	• abnormal androgen secretion • abnormal gonadotropin secretion • abnormal prolactin secretion
cervical abnormalities	• abnormal Pap smears • fetal DES exposure • mucus *(postcoital test)*
sperm disorders	<u>no sperm:</u> • Klinefelter's • ductal obstruction • varicocele <u>few sperm:</u> • genetic • maturation arrest • heat <u>abnormal morphology:</u> • infections (mumps) <u>abnormal motility:</u> • infections (mumps) • immunologic incompatibility

***Overall causes*:**
50% women
30% men
20% combination of the two

229

15.9.) <u>NIPPLE DISCHARGE</u>

Nipple discharge is common and often harmless. However it can be a first sign of ductal carcinomas and should be investigated carefully. The nature of the discharge may give a clue but does not allow diagnosis.

benign epithelial debris	• thick, grayish • common in middle-aged parous women
breast abscess	• thick, purulent
breast cancer	• bloody or watery • sometimes purulent
milky	• choriocarcinoma ➢ phenothiazines ➢ reserpine ➢ cimetidine ➢ oral contraceptives

Most common cause of bloody nipple discharge:
benign intraductal papilloma!

15.10.) BREAST CANCER

Breast cancer is the most common cancer in women and has the second highest mortality (after lung cancer). Fibrocystic change is very common and benign.

FIBROCYSTIC CHANGE	BREAST CANCER
• often bilateral • multiple nodules • menstrual variation • may regress during pregnancy	• often unilateral • single mass • no cyclic variations

 Fibrocystic change does not increase risk of breast cancer, but makes detection more difficult.

PERHAPS BENIGN	PERHAPS MALIGNANT
• discrete, smooth • movable • tender	• ill-defined, thickened • non-movable • edema
Mammogram: • round, ovoid, smooth • clearly defined margins • may contain calcifications	Mammogram: • distinct, irregular tumor mass • projection of dense spicules • may contain calcifications

---

RISK FACTORS:
(1.) family history
(2.) age of patient
(3.) estrogens

15.11.) <u>OVARIAN CANCER</u>

Second most common gynecological malignancy (after endometrial cancer). Unfortunately it is often diagnosed too late…

Stage I	confined to 1 or 2 ovaries
Stage II	pelvic spread
Stage III	intra-abdominal spread
Stage IV	distant spread

<u>RISK FACTORS:</u>
(1.) family history of cancer
(2.) nulliparity
(3.) infertility
(4.) late child bearing
(5.) late menopause
(6.) diet rich in animal fats

 Most common presentation: vague abdominal complaints.

15.12.) <u>ENDOMETRIAL CANCER</u>

Most common gynecological malignancy, affecting mostly elderly women.
Postmenopausal bleeding should always be investigated very carefully
(D&C or endometrial biopsy with an aspiration device).

Stage I	limited to **endometrium**
Stage II	involves endocervical **glands or stroma**
Stage III	invades **serosa** or involves **vagina** or pelvic and/or paraaortic lymph nodes
Stage IV	involves **rectum or bladder** or distant metastases

<u>RISK FACTORS:</u>
(1.) obesity
(2.) nulliparity
(3.) estrogen use
(4.) pelvic radiation

Most common presentation: abnormal uterine bleeding.

15.13.) <u>VAGINAL DISCHARGE</u>

Vaginal discharge is due to infections and the color and smell of the discharge gives important clues for diagnosis:

Candida	• white, curd-like • sweet odor
Chlamydia	• yellow, mucopurulent • odorless
Trichomonas	• frothy, greenish • foul smelling
Gardnerella	• green/gray • foul smelling **clue cells:** epithelial cells with cocci **whiff test:** add KOH to discharge → fishy smell
Gonorrhea	**in 80%:** asymptomatic **in 20%:** yellowish green discharge from Bartholin's glands

15.14.) CERVICITIS / STDS

Chlamydia is the most common STD in the US. If undiagnosed and untreated, these diseases cause chronic pelvic inflammatory disease and reduce fertility.

	SIGNS & SYMPTOMS	DIAGNOSIS
chlamydia	• often asymptomatic • or cervicitis	• culture
gonorrhea	• asymptomatic • or purulent discharge	• culture (Thayer-Martin)
syphilis	• chancre sore • fever • skin rash (secondary)	• VDRL • FTAbs
herpes	• multiple tender vesicles • fever (if primary)	
chancroid	• soft, painful ulcer	• biopsy
human papilloma virus	• warts • painless	

PELVIC INFLAMMATORY DISEASE:
(1.) cervicitis (often asymptomatic)
(2.) salpingitis (often also few symptoms)
   → risk of ectopic pregnancy
(3.) peritoneal adhesions (uterus, adnexa)
   →dyspareunia, infertility, chronic pelvic pain

15.15.) CERVIX CANCER

Cervix cancer is considered a "sexually transmitted cancer" and strongly associated with human papilloma virus infection (types 16,18, 31, 33 and 35). Annual Pap smear for all sexually active women is the most important preventive measure.

Stage I	carcinoma limited to **cervix**
Stage II	involvement of **upper 2/3 vagina** or involvement of parametria
Stage III	involvement of **lower 1/3 vagina** or involvement of pelvic sidewall
Stage IV	involvement of **bladder or rectum** or distant metastases

RISK FACTORS:
(1.) multiple sex partners at early age
(2.) human papilloma virus
(3.) smoking

15.16.) <u>PAP SMEAR</u>

BETHESDA CLASSIFICATION:

benign cellular changes	1. infections:
	  • Trichomonas infection
	  • Candida infection
	
	2. reactive changes:
	  • inflammation
	  • atrophic vaginitis

epithelial cell abnormalities	3. atypical squamous cells of undetermined significance:
	(borderline between severe reactive change and mild dysplasia)
	
	4. low-grade intraepithelial lesion:
	  • human papilloma virus
	  • mild dysplasia (CIN 1)
	
	5. high-grade intraepithelial lesion:
	  • moderate dysplasia (CIN 2)
	  • severe dysplasia (CIN 3)
	  • carcinoma in situ
	
	6. squamous cell carcinoma

> **False negative rate of Pap smear: 15 - 30%**

An abnormal Pap smear requires follow-up: either a colposcopic biopsy or a loop excision (cervical conization).

PRIMARY AMENORRHEA
➢ If uterus absent: karyotype
➢ If uterus present and vagina patent: workup like secondary amenorrhea

SECONDARY AMENORRHEA
➢ Rule out pregnancy!
➢ If hirsutism present: rule out polycystic ovaries, ovarian and adrenal tumors
➢ Progesterone challenge and FSH to distinguish between hypothalamic and gonadal failure
➢ Prolactinoma: transsphenoidal destruction of pituitary adenoma.
    Induce ovulation with bromocriptine

DYSMENORRHEA
➢ NSAIDs (ibuprofen)
➢ Oral contraceptives → anovulation → decreased prostaglandin production
➢ Adenomyosis and endometriosis may require surgical treatment

INFERTILITY
➢ **Male factor:** semen analysis, postcoital test, consider removal of varicocele, consider sperm aspiration and IVF
➢ **Ovarian factor:** document ovulation (basal temperature, progesterone levels), induce with clomiphene, bromocriptine for anovulation due to prolactin excess.
➢ **Cervical factor:** treat chronic infections, mucus quality, test behavior of sperms in mucus, consider steroids if antisperm antibodies present
➢ **Tubal factor:** determine patency, consider *in vitro fertilization*
➢ **Uterine factor:** treat endometritis, consider removal of myomas

POLYCYSTIC OVARIES
➢ Weight loss
➢ Clomiphene to induce ovulation
➢ Ovarian wedge resection rarely necessary
➢ Endometrial biopsies to exclude cancer

TOXIC SHOCK SYNDROME

➢ Aggressive supportive therapy: Fluid and electrolytes, antibiotics
➢ Monitor urine output and pulmonary wedge pressure
➢ Consider replacement of coagulation factors
➢ Causes of death:
  1. respiratory distress syndrome
  2. cardiovascular failure
  3. hemorrhage (DIC)

ENDOMETRIOSIS

Medical therapy: suppress ovarian function and endometrial growth
➢ **Induce "pseudopregnancy":** maintain high progesterone levels
  (side-effects: depression, constipation, weight gain, breakthrough bleeding)
➢ **Induce "pseudomenopause":** reduce estrogen and progesterone levels
  - danazol (weak androgen) suppresses gonadotropin release

Surgical therapy: preserve fertility if possible
➢ Laparoscopy: laser or electrocoagulation
➢ For intractable pelvic pain: hysterectomy+ salpingo-oophorectomy
                    followed by estrogen replacement therapy

PELVIC INFLAMMATORY DISEASE

➢ Empiric antibiotic treatment (ceftriaxone plus doxycycline)
➢ Hospitalize if temperature >102.2 °F or signs of peritonitis (guarding, rebound tenderness) are present
➢ Examine and treat all male partners (if you can find them)

BARTHOLIN'S GLAND ABSCESS

➢ Simple incision and drainage provides temporary relief

FIBROCYSTIC CHANGE

- **FNA:** clear fluid: observe. Residual mass or bloody: excisional biopsy
- Avoid trauma
- Giving up coffee and tea often helps

FIBROADENOMA

- Excision under local anesthesia

BREAST CANCER

- **Lumpectomy + axillary lymph node resection:** option for tumors < 5cm
- **Simple mastectomy:** breast removal, lymph nodes left in place
- **Modified radical mastectomy:** removal of breast, pectoralis major fascia (but not muscle) and lymph nodes
- **Radical mastectomy:** en-bloc removal of breast, pectoral muscles and axillary nodes

- Adjuvant chemotherapy if axillary lymph nodes positive
- Tamoxifen if estrogen receptor positive

OVARIAN CANCER
➢ Surgery: hysterectomy + bilateral salpingo-oophorectomy
➢ Adjuvant chemotherapy
➢ Dysgerminomas: combination chemotherapy or radiotherapy

UTERINE LEIOMYOMA
➢ If asymptomatic or patient postmenopause: no treatment necessary
➢ Consider removal if excessively large (>12 weeks uterus)

ENDOMETRIAL CANCER
➢ Hysterectomy + bilateral salpingo-oophorectomy
Advanced stage:
➢ Give progesterone
➢ Adjuvant chemotherapy (doxorubicin, cisplatin) or radiotherapy

ABNORMAL PAP SMEAR
➢ If Class II or above → colposcopy-directed biopsy
➢ If biopsy inconclusive → cone biopsy (LEEP)

CERVIX CANCER
➢ Early stage: radical hysterectomy
➢ Late stage: radiation therapy plus chemotherapy

OBSTETRICS

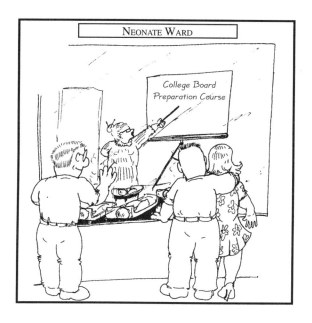

16.1.) <u>DRUG USE DURING PREGNANCY</u>

	SAFE	UNSAFE
hypertension	β-blockers	thiazides ACE inhibitors
diabetes	insulin	sulfonylureas
asthma	cromolyn terbutaline	steroids
analgesics	acetaminophen	ibuprofen indomethacin
antibiotics	penicillins sulfonamides erythromycin amphotericin B	quinine tetracyclines
anticoagulants	heparin	warfarin

<u>Some common drugs to avoid</u>
<u>during breast feeding:</u>
- ➤ antineoplastic agents
- ➤ bromocriptine
- ➤ cimetidine
- ➤ ergotamines
- ➤ gold salts
- ➤ lithium
- ➤ thiouracil

 Do not breast feed with HIV, chronic HBV or CMV infection!

16.2.) PARITY

Some definitions you need to know when taking an obstetric history:

nulligravida	• is not and never has been pregnant
primigravida	• is or has been pregnant • irrespective of pregnancy outcome
nullipara	• has never completed a pregnancy • may or may not have aborted
primipara	• has completed one pregnancy (> 500g , dead or alive)
multipara	• has completed two or more pregnancies

 A women with her first triplets is also primipara!

16.3.) <u>PREGNANCY SIGNS</u>

presumptive signs	**menses > 10 days late**
	morning nausea: occurs at 4-6 weeks of gestation
	breast changes: tenderness enlargement of Montgomery's tubercles
	chloasma: darkening of skin over forehead, bridge of nose and cheekbones
	quickening: first perception of fetal movement occurs at 16-20 weeks
probable signs	**uterus enlarged:** 12 weeks: above symphysis 20 weeks: at umbilicus
	Hegar's sign: softening of cervix
	Chadwick's sign: bluish discoloration of cervix
	hCG or β-hCG
certain signs	**fetal heart tones:** 17-19 weeks by auscultation
	ultrasound identification: possible after 6 weeks

 Nägele's rule : *9 month plus 7 days from beginning of LMP.*

246

16.4.) <u>PREGNANCY SCREENS</u>

initial workup	• hemoglobin • blood group, Rh factor • rubella titers • syphilis (VDRL) • Pap smear **if at risk:** HBV, HIV, toxoplasmosis

urine test	• if bacteriuria (> 105/ml): treat!
	  (even if asymptomatic)
	
	• glucosuria is common!
	  (not important if blood sugar is normal)

at 16 weeks	<u>Triple screen (Down syndrome)</u> • AFP + hCG + estriol • if abnormal → amniocentesis
amniocentesis	• offer to all women > 35 years • previous chromosomal abnormality • history of spontaneous abortions ○ usually done between 16-18th week ○ < 1% risk of fetal loss
chorionic villi sample	○ best done between 9th -11th week ○ 5% risk of fetal loss

AFP elevated:	- open neural tube - multiple gestation - duodenal atresia
AFP decreased:	- Down syndrome

16.5.) PREGNANCY BLEEDING

Different causes of bleeding at different times of pregnancy:

first trimester	<ul><li>very common</li><li>50% result in spontaneous abortion</li><li>50% continue as normal pregnancy</li></ul>
second trimester	<ul><li>low lying placenta</li></ul>
third trimester	**bloody show:** mixed with mucus, labor **placenta previa:** heavy, painless bleeding [1] **abruptio placentae:** none or heavy bleeding continuous abdominal pain sustained uterine contraction fetal distress DIC **uterus rupture:** sudden cessation of uterine contractions disappearance of fetal heart tones
puerperium	up to 500 ml blood loss is normal <ul><li>hypotonic uterus [2]</li><li>ruptured uterus</li><li>retention of placental tissue</li><li>trauma (lacerations, episiotomy)</li></ul>

[1] *do not palpate cervix unless ready for delivery!*
[2] *common if general anesthesia is used (try to massage uterus or give oxytocin).*

Kleihauer-Betke test:
fetal RBCs are more resistant to alkaline pH than maternal RBCs.

16.6.) PREGNANCY COMPLICATIONS

gestational diabetes	• glucosuria often due to increased GFR • Glucola: 1h oral glucose tolerance test **Increased risk of:** (1.) preeclampsia (2.) hyaline membrane disease (3.) large infants (4.) infections ➢ *diet or insulin*
hypertension	• 140/90 or more than 30 mmHg systolic rise • in early pregnancy: suggests mole ➢ *hospitalization, bed rest*
preeclampsia	• hypertension plus proteinuria • more common in nullipara ➢ *hydralazine, Mg^{2+}-sulfate (anticonvulsive)* ➢ *delivery*
eclampsia	• preeclampsia plus convulsions
patients with pre-existing heart disease (see 4.14)	**Class I or II:** can go through pregnancy **Class III:** may be indication for abortion deliver vaginal if possible **Class IV:** high mortality due to cardiac failure

16.7.) <u>SPONTANEOUS ABORTION</u>

It is estimated that about 50% of all conceptions are aborted spontaneously!

early abortion	• often unnoticed • usually due to chromosomal abnormalities
threatened abortion	• **no cervical dilation** o bleeding o uterine cramping
inevitable abortion	• **ruptured membranes** • **cervix dilated** o bleeding o uterine cramping
incomplete abortion	• **retained placental tissue**
missed abortion	• **no labor or passage of tissue** o death of fetus or embryo
habitual abortion	• three or more spontaneous abortions

<u>Causes of habitual abortion:</u>
(1.) defective zygote
(2.) cervical incompetence
(3.) infections
(4.) hormonal dysfunction
(5.) chromosomal abnormalities

16.8.) <u>LABOR</u>

	TRUE LABOR	FALSE LABOR
intervals	regular	irregular
contraction	intensity increases gradually	intensity constant
sedation	does not affect contractions	stops contractions

first stage	<ul><li>about 12 hours (primipara)</li><li>cervix effacement and dilation</li></ul>**latent phase:** slow dilation of cervix **active phase:** dilation > 1.2 cm/h
second stage	<ul><li>about 1 hour (primipara)</li><li>delivery of infant</li></ul>
third stage	<ul><li>within 5 min.</li><li>delivery of placenta</li></ul>

Indications for induction of labor:
- ruptured membranes > 48h
- chorioamnionitis

<u>Stations are measured in cm below level of ischial spine:</u>
O station   = engagement
+1 station = presenting part 1 cm below ischial spine
+2 station = presenting part 2 cm below ischial spine
.
.
.

16.9.) <u>LABOR PATTERNS</u>

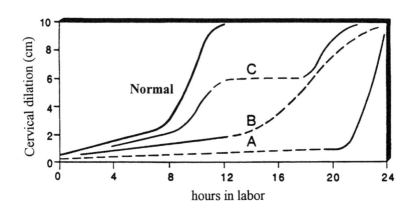

From *Obstetrics and Gynecology*, 2nd edition, p. 190, by C.R.B. Beckmann et al.
Copyright 1995 by Williams & Wilkins, Baltimore, MD. Used with permission.

- **A:** prolonged latent phase
- **B:** prolonged active phase
- **C:** arrest of active phase

<u>PREMATURE RUPTURE OF MEMBRANES</u>

- danger of chorioamnionitis
- amniotic fluid shows ferning
- amniotic fluid has pH > 7.0 (Nitrazine test)

- amniotic band syndrome: - fetus becomes entangled in membranes
  - resulting in deformities, finger amputations...

16.10.) <u>PREMATURITY</u>

- **Immature:** gestational age 20-28 weeks
- **Premature:** gestational age 28-37 weeks
  (irrespective of birth weight or fetal maturity)

RISK FACTORS: - African-Americans
　　　　　　　　　 - low socioeconomic status
　　　　　　　　　 - previous premature births
　　　　　　　　　 - **smoking**

- Monitor risk patients: weekly cervical exams

- **Cervical incompetence:**　history of second trimester abortions in
　　　　　　　　　　　　　　absence of uterine contractions

- **L/S ratio** preferably > 2

16.11.) <u>POSTMATURITY</u>

- **Gestational age 42 weeks or more**
  (irrespective of birth weight or fetal maturity)

- **Signs of dysmaturity:**　dry, wrinkled skin, loss of subcutaneous fat,
　　　　　　　　　　　　　meconium staining, long nails

nonstress test	- 3 or more fetal movements in 30 min - heart rate accelerations > 15 beats/min
oxytocin stress test	**negative:** no or early deceleration **positive:** late decelerations
biophysical profile (ultrasound)	1. nonstress test 2. fetal breathing, 3. tone and 4. motion 5. amount of amniotic fluid

253

16.12.) <u>THE FETUS</u>

Distinguish between lie, presentation and position:

fetal lie	long axis of fetus in relation to long axis of uterus • longitudinal • transverse • oblique

fetal presentation	portion of fetus that can be felt through cervix
	
	cephalic: vertex
	                face
	                brow
	
	frank breech (thighs are flexed, legs are extended)
	
	complete breech (thighs are flexed, legs are flexed)
	
	footling breech

fetal position	relation of fetal occiput[1] to maternal birth canal • left occiput anterior • left occiput transverse • left occiput posterior etc....

[1] *or chin in case of face presentation.*

 Most common is longitudinal lie, cephalic presentation, occiput anterior.

16.13.) <u>FETAL HEART RATE</u>

normal	• good variability (120 to 160 beats/min)
absent variability	• **high perinatal mortality!**
early decelerations	• not a/w poor fetal outcome • not caused by hypoxemia
late decelerations	• **fetal hypoxemia** • myocardial compression a/w hypertension, preeclampsia, maternal hypotension, excessive uterine contractions (oxytocin)
variable decelerations	• transient compression of umbilical cord

From *Obstetrics and Gynecology*, 2nd edition, p. 201, by C.R.B. Beckmann et al.
Copyright 1995 by Williams & Wilkins, Baltimore, MD. Used with permission.

<u>Management of late decelerations:</u>
→ if late decelerations persist sample fetal scalp blood and monitor pH.
→ if pH < 7.25 repeat every 30 min.
→ if pH < 7.20 deliver!

16.14.) <u>ANESTHESIA</u>

paracervical block	• relieves pain from uterine contractions • not sufficient for labor • *may cause fetal bradycardia*
pudendal block	• **for spontaneous delivery** • for repair of episiotomy • not sufficient for forceps delivery • *may cause systemic toxicity*
epidural anesthesia	• **for vaginal delivery or c-section** • not always effective analgesia (not enough for perineum) • *inadvertent subarachnoid blockade may cause systemic and CNS toxicity*
spinal anesthesia (subarachnoid)	• **for vaginal delivery or c-section** <u>COMPARED TO EPIDURAL</u>: ○ more rapid onset ○ less fetal toxicity ○ higher risk of severe maternal hypotension
general anesthesia	• **for emergencies or if spinal/epidural are contraindicated** **NO_2**: - does not interfere with uterine contractions - does not prolong labor **halothane**: may cause atonic uterus → hemorrhage

If hemorrhage or coagulation disorders are present, spinal and epidural anesthesia are contraindicated.

16.15.) EPISIOTOMY

	MIDLINE	MEDIOLATERAL
advantages	• easy to repair • small blood loss • minimal post-op. pain • rare dyspareunia	• more space for breech deliveries
disadvantages	• may extend (into anal sphincter)	• more difficult to repair • greater blood loss • commonly post-op. pain • dyspareunia

16.16.) <u>TROPHOBLASTIC DISEASE</u>

HYDATIDIFORM MOLE	CHORIOCARCINOMA
<ul><li>diffuse hydropic chorionic villi</li><li>hyperplastic trophoblasts</li></ul><ul><li>vaginal bleeding</li><li>uterine size greater than date</li><li>hyperemesis</li></ul><ul><li>**invasive mole:** invades myometrium</li></ul>➤ high β-hCG	<ul><li>proliferation of cytotrophoblast</li><li>proliferation of syncytiotrophoblast</li><li>no villi present</li></ul>**following molar pregnancy** **following spontaneous abortion** **following term pregnancy** ➤ high β-hCG

<u>COMPLETE MOLE</u>:
- empty oocyte fertilized by sperm
- 46XX (both X are paternal origin)

<u>INCOMPLETE MOLE</u>:
- mole plus fetal remnants
- triploid set of chromosomes

HYPEREMESIS

➤ Small frequent meals (light and dry)
➤ High dose vit. B6 may help
➤ Use antinausea drugs only as last resort
➤ Hospitalize if patient becomes dehydrated and ketonuric

GESTATIONAL DIABETES

➤ Glucosuria is unreliable finding
➤ Glucola (50g sugar) screening test
➤ Diet and exercise
➤ Close monitoring of blood glucose and fetal growth
➤ Glucose tolerance usually returns to normal postpartum, but 50% risk of diabetes mellitus in the future

PREECLAMPSIA

➤ Hospitalize!
➤ Monitor proteinuria
➤ Monitor fetus. Give corticosteroids to accelerate lung maturation
➤ Past 28 weeks, if preeclampsia is severe: deliver!
➤ Anticonvulsants (Mg^{2+} sulfate) during labor

ECLAMPSIA

➤ Seizures: Mg^{2+} sulfate or phenytoin
➤ Hypertension: hydralazine or labetalol
➤ Attempt labor. If eclampsia is severe → cesarean section!

ABRUPTIO PLACENTAE

(if concealed behind placenta: bleeding may not apparent!)
- ➤ Rupture membranes and prepare delivery
- ➤ If fetus is dead or questionable → vaginal delivery
- ➤ If placenta separation is limited → vaginal delivery
- ➤ If hemorrhage uncontrollable (maternal indication) → c-section
- ➤ If fetus viable but under distress (fetal indication) → c-section

PLACENTA PREVIA

- ➤ Avoid vaginal examination
- ➤ Confirm or rule out by ultrasound
- ➤ Cesarean section

PREMATURE RUPTURE OF MEMBRANES

- ➤ If gestational age > 33 weeks → deliver to reduce risk of amnionitis
- ➤ If gestational age < 33 weeks → determine fetal lung maturity. Give corticosteroids to accelerate maturation. Closely monitor patient for signs of infection
- ➤ If gestational age <26 weeks → little hope for fetal survival

ECTOPIC PREGNANCY

- ➤ Culdocentesis: non-clotting blood indicates bleeding from ruptured ectopic gestation
- ➤ Exploratory laparoscopy. If bleeding is profound: laparotomy

PREMATURE LABOR
- Emergency: tocolytic agents (terbutaline), $MgSO_4$
- Continued care: oral β-sympathomimetics

INCOMPETENT CERVIX
- Rule out preterm labor!
- Prophylactic cerclage may be placed at 12-16 weeks

PROLONGED LABOR
- Exclude fetopelvic disproportion
- Supportive measures
- Avoid excessive sedation or regional anesthesia
- Avoid oxytocin if contractions are already adequate

HYDATIDIFORM MOLE
- Dilation and suction
- Sharp curettage
- Hysterectomy not necessary
- Monitor β-hCG for 6-12 months

CHORIOCARCINOMA
- Chemotherapy
- Cure rate almost 100%
- Future pregnancies possible

POSTPARTUM HEMORRHAGE

➤ Uterine atony: try massage first.
➤ If massage doesn't work: methylergonovine, oxytocin or PGF2α
➤ Rule out uterus inversion (requires immediate manual replacement)

POSTPARTUM SEPSIS

(temperature > 100.4°F within first 24h after delivery)
➤ Common causes: *Chlamydia*, *Bacteroides*, *Mycoplasma*
➤ Bed rest (semi-Fowler position), antibiotics

POSTPARTUM DEPRESSION

➤ Occurs most commonly between days 3 and 10 postpartum
➤ Should be treated if lasting >72 hours, or if patient is suicidal or psychotic

POSTPARTUM THROMBOPHLEBITIS

➤ Early ambulation is important
➤ Consider prophylaxis for phlebothrombosis
➤ Advise not to use oral contraceptives
➤ Advise to stop smoking

PEDIATRICS

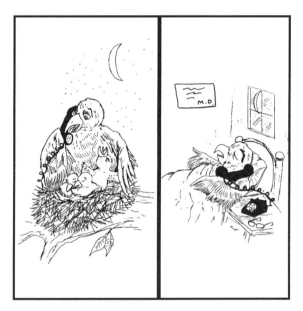

"Just keep feeding them on demand, Mrs. Rogers.
Some children need more than others."

17.1.) <u>BIRTH TRAUMA</u> - 1

Head trauma during delivery is more likely when the mother has a small pelvis or if the infant is large for gestational age. Consider C-section rather than attempting difficult versions or vacuum or high-forceps deliveries!

Here is the range of trauma, from mild to severe:

caput succedaneum	• diffuse edema of scalp soft tissue • **not limited to area of bones**
cephalhematoma	• subperiosteal hemorrhage • **limited to area of affected bone**
subdural hemorrhage	• **mechanical trauma, forceps** (cephalopelvic disproportion) • *more common in <u>large</u> infants*
periventricular hemorrhage **intraventricular hemorrhage**	• **often occurs without obvious trauma** • vulnerability to cerebral blood flow and pressure changes • *occurs in <u>small or preterm</u> infants* • hypotension, bradycardia, apnea • lethargy, seizures, coma

17.2.) <u>BIRTH TRAUMA</u> - <u>2</u>

A) <u>INJURIES TO BRACHIAL PLEXUS</u>:

Erb-Duchenne	injury of <u>superior</u> brachial plexus (C5, C6) • due to lateral pull of head during shoulder extraction • **"waiter's tip" position** (forearm extended and internally rotated, wrist flexed) • absent biceps reflex
Klumpke	injury of <u>inferior</u> brachial plexus (C8, T1) • wrist drop • Horner's syndrome[1] common

[1] *ptosis, miosis and dry, red skin on half side of face*

B) <u>OTHER INJURIES</u>:

clavicle fracture	• usually "green-stick" • initially often asymptomatic
amnion band syndrome	• a/w early rupture of membranes • loss of a digit or limb due to constriction

17.3.) APGAR SCORE

In 1958 Apgar developed a scoring system to describe the neurologic status and cardiorespiratory adaptation to birth. You need to know the 5 components and be able to calculate the score when given a case presentation on the USMLE.

	0	1	2
heart rate	none	< 100/min	> 100/min
respiratory effort	none	slow, irregular	good, crying
muscle tone	limp	some flexion	active motion
reflex irritability	absent	grimace	cough or sneeze
color	blue, pale	acrocyanosis	pink

reproduced with permission from: Apgar et al., JAMA 168:1985-88, 1958

 - 7 or above after 5 min. is good.

- If the score remains 3 or less for more than 10 min. there will be an increased risk of cerebral palsy.

17.4.) <u>SUBSTANCE ABUSE DURING PREGNANCY</u>

Substance abuse during pregnancy has severe effects on the fetus:

heroin, PCP	• no congenital abnormalities **<u>Neonatal withdrawal</u>:** • jitteriness • hyperreflexia • seizures
cocaine	• risk of placenta abruption • increased risk for SIDS
inhalants	• neurotoxicity • microcephaly
tobacco	• increased frequency of abortion • low birth weight

Testing maternal urine for drugs requires consent!
Testing infant's blood or urine for drugs does not require consent!

17.5.) <u>TERATOGENS</u>

Teratogens are drugs or toxins that interfere with the development of fetal organs. The critical period is between the 3rd and 8th week of conception, when the organs are being formed. Earlier exposure either kills the embryo or has on effect at all. Later exposure is more likely to interfere with growth and function.

alcohol	• microphthalmia • short palpebral fissures o flat nasal bridge o broad upper lip
retinoids	• severe CNS abnormalities o congenital heart defects o ear malformations (small or absent)
diphenylhydantoin	• hypoplasia of distal phalanges • small nails o flat nasal bridge o cleft lip/palate
warfarin	• chondrodysplasia (stippled vertebral and femoral epiphyses) o nasal hypoplasia
thalidomide	• upper limb phocomelia • lower limb phocomelia

Retinoic acid cream (for treatment of acne) should also be avoided during pregnancy, even though its systemic concentration is probably too low to be teratogenic.

17.6.) CONGENITAL INFECTIONS

toxoplasmosis	**T** **O**	• hydrocephalus • **generalized calcifications** • chorioretinitis
rubella	**R**	• heart defects • microcephaly, microphthalmia • **cataracts** • **hearing loss**
CMV	**C**	• microcephaly, microphthalmia • **periventricular calcifications** • chorioretinitis
herpes	**H**	• microphthalmia • retinopathy • intracranial calcifications
syphilis		**newborns often asymptomatic** **after 3-12 weeks:** • jaundice • hemolytic anemia • rhinitis ("snuffles") • rash on palms and soles **permanent stigma:** • Hutchinson's teeth • saddle nose • saber shins
varicella		• **limb hypoplasia** • cutaneous scars • cortical atrophy

17.7.) <u>TRISOMIES</u>

Loss of an autosomal chromosome is not compatible with life. Trisomies (except for 21) are also lethal:

	FEATURES	LIFE EXPECTANCY	PRENATAL SURVIVAL	RECURRENCE RISK
trisomy 21	• congenital heart defects • mongoloid eye slant • depressed nasal bridge • protruding tongue • transverse palmar crease	50% live > 50 years (early Alzheimer's)	25% [1]	about 1% [2]
trisomy 18	• clenched hands • overlapping 2nd and 5th finger • low set ears • short sternum • nail hypoplasia	90% die in first month	5%	< 1%
trisomy 13	• severe CNS abnormalities • microphthalmia • polydactyly • cleft lip / palate	100% lethal by 6 months	1%	< 1%

[1] *i.e. 75% are spontaneously aborted.*   [2] *recurrence risk is much higher if due to translocation!*

17.8.) <u>MULTIFACTORIAL BIRTH DEFECTS</u>

These are common defects with many, often non-specific causes:

cleft lip / cleft palate	• cleft lip (with or without cleft palate) is genetically distinct form isolated cleft palate.
anencephaly **spina bifida**	• a/w folate deficiency
congenital heart defects	• common component of many syndromes.

 Folate supplementation (1 mg/day) reduces neural tube defects and is recommended for all pregnant women! This is usually combined with iron supplementation to prevent anemia of pregnancy.

17.9.) <u>PERINATAL VIRAL INFECTIONS</u>

Perinatal infections occur near term and are transmitted to the fetus by the mother. Do not confuse with **congenital infections** (17.6), which occur during early pregnancy and leave specific birth defects!

varicella	**if mother infected within days of delivery:** • may be severe, disseminated • often fatal encephalitis ➢ *give immunoglobulin after birth*
herpes simplex	• **high risk if primary maternal infection** • low risk if recurrent maternal infection • herpetic encephalitis ➢ *c-section if active lesions are present*
hepatitis B	• usually results in chronic subclinical hepatitis • rarely fulminant hepatitis ➢ *screen all pregnant women for HBsAg* ➢ *c-section not necessary* ➢ *give immunoglobulin after birth*
HIV [1]	**typical onset of symptoms 4-6 months after birth:** • lymphadenopathy • hepatomegaly • splenomegaly • failure to thrive ➢ *c-section not helpful (transplacental transfer of HIV!)* ➢ *AZT*

[1] *IgG antibodies in < 9 month old infant may be of maternal origin!*

272

17.10.) RESPIRATORY DISTRESS SYNDROME

Also known as *hyaline membrane disease*, is due to lack of surfactant, a mixture of phospholipids made by type II pneumocytes.

risk factors	• male sex • premature birth • second born twin • perinatal asphyxia • maternal diabetes • L/S ratio < 2
clinical features	• tachypnea • nasal flaring • grunting • cyanosis • "ground glass" appearance on CXR
complications	<u>intrinsic:</u> • pneumothorax • pulmonary emphysema <u>oxygen therapy:</u> • bronchopulmonary dysplasia • retinopathy

17.11.) MECONIUM ASPIRATION SYNDROME

Some meconium staining of amniotic fluid is seen in up to 15% of normal pregnancies

risk factors	• meconium is passed during intrauterine stress • more common in post term infants
clinical features	• cyanosis, tachypnea • persistent pulmonary hypertension

17.12.) <u>NEONATAL CONJUNCTIVITIS</u>

chemical irritation	• **within first 2 days after birth** • due to silver nitrate
gonorrhea	• **1 to 2 weeks after birth** • prevent with silver nitrate or erythromycin drops instilled into each eye after delivery (recommended for every newborn!)
chlamydia	• **1 to 2 weeks after birth** • watch for systemic infection (i.e. pneumonia)
viral	• **in infants > 3 months** • usually adenovirus

<u>Symptoms:</u>
(1.) purulent discharge
(2.) eye lid reddening or swelling

Mucous drainage from eye for 1-2 days after birth is normal and does not indicate conjunctivitis!

Constant tearing after birth may indicate a blockage of the nasolacrimal duct.

17.13.) <u>NEONATAL HYPERBILIRUBINEMIA</u>

	UC	C	
physiologic jaundice	X		• 3 to 5 days postnatal • due to increased bilirubin production and relatively immature liver
breast milk jaundice	X		• 2 to 3 weeks after birth • due to increased bilirubin absorption *brief interruption of breast feeding (usually not necessary)*
hemolysis	X		• Rh, ABO incompatibility • spherocytosis • G6PDH deficiency
enzyme defects	X		**Gilbert (mild)** (decreased hepatic bilirubin uptake) **Crigler-Najjar (severe)** (deficient glucuronyl transferase)
		X	**Dubin Johnson** (impaired hepatocellular secretion)
cholestasis		X	• bile duct stenosis • biliary atresia • hepatitis • cystic fibrosis
kernicterus	X		• unconjugated bilirubin > 20 mg/dl • staining of basal ganglia • lethargy, hypotonia, encephalopathy

UC: *mainly unconjugated bilirubin*   **C**: *mainly conjugated bilirubin*

17.14.) <u>SMALL & LARGE INFANTS</u>

The size and weight of the infant must always be related to gestational age.

SGA: Small for gestational age
AGA: Appropriate for gestational age
LGA: Large for gestational age

<u>COMMON CAUSES:</u>

SGA	LGA
2 SD below expected	2 SD above expected
• chromosomal abnormalities • TORCH o alcohol, drug abuse o maternal hypertension o placenta insufficiency	• diabetic mother • genetic/ racial • Prader Willi

Low birthweight infant: *< 2500 g at birth*
(can be SGA, AGA or LGA)

<u>PROBLEMS OF INFANTS OF DIABETIC MOTHERS:</u>
(1.) birth trauma
(2.) hypoglycemia
(3.) respiratory distress syndrome

- L/S ratio is not reliable for infants of diabetic mothers!
- better: amniotic fluid phosphatidyl glycerin.

17.15.) <u>NUTRITION</u>

breast milk [1]	**Compared to cow milk:** • more fat • more carbohydrates • more lactalbumin, less casein o both lack Vit. D !
supplementation	<u>Iron:</u> • start supplementation at age 4-6 months (earlier in preterm infants) <u>Fluoride:</u> • for all breast fed infants • or if Fl⁻ content of drinking water is poor <u>Calcium, Vit. D:</u> • for breast fed infants at risk (lack of sunlight) <u>Vit. B12:</u> • for breast fed infants if mother is vegetarian
commercial formulas	**cow milk based (with added whey protein)** <u>Soy protein formulas:</u> • "hypoallergenic", but cross-reactivity is common • useful after diarrhea (transient lactase deficiency)

[1] *10% weight loss by 2 weeks is normal for breast fed infants.*

 Human milk is best for humans; cow milk is best for calves.

<u>Viruses that can be transmitted via breast milk:</u>
➢ hepatitis B
➢ HIV
➢ rubella
➢ herpes
➢ CMV

17.16.) <u>GROWTH CURVES</u>

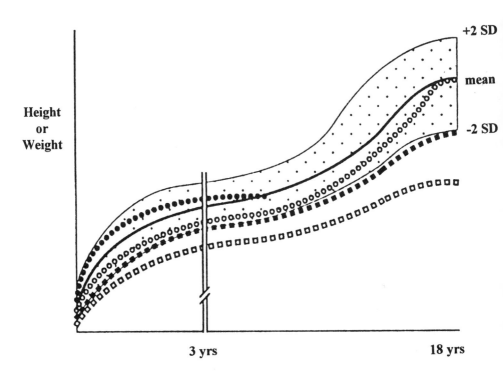

Height
or
Weight

+2 SD

mean

-2 SD

3 yrs   18 yrs

From *Rudolph's Pediatrics*, 20th edition, page 4, edited by A.M. Rudolph.
Copyright 1996 by Appleton & Lange. Used with permission.

Postnatal-onset pathologic growth ●
Constitutional growth delay   ○
Genetic short stature   ■
Prenatal-onset pathologic growth   □

278

17.17.) <u>INFECTIOUS DISEASES OF CHILDHOOD</u>

rubeola (measles)	• 8 to 12 days incubation • **3 to 5 days prodromal** **(cough, coryza, conjunctivitis)** • followed by **Koplik's spots** • then maculopapular rash neck → face → arms → trunk • subacute sclerosing panencephalitis (rare but deadly complication)
rubella (German measles)	• 14 to 21 days incubation • **mild prodrome, tender lymph nodes** • maculopapular rash, 3 day fever neck → face → arms → trunk • infection during first trimester results in 30% chance of congenital abnormalities
roseola (exanthema subitum)	• acute high fever • **maculopapular rash as fever falls** • rash begins on trunk

17.18.) <u>INFECTIOUS DISEASES OF CHILDHOOD</u>

varicella (chickenpox)	• 11 to 21 days incubation • mild prodrome, anorexia • **generalized pruritic vesicles** • begin on trunk → face, extremities • lesions at different stages of healing *patients with herpes zoster can transmit* *virus to susceptible children!*
fifth disease (erythema infectiosum)	• 7 days incubation • no prodrome, no fever • sudden bright rash **"slapped cheeks"**, then maculopapular rash on trunk and extremities • complication: aplastic anemia
scarlet fever	• 1 to 7 days incubation • pharyngitis • rapid onset fever, headache, vomiting • **"sand paper" rash** • **starts at time of fever** • **spares the face** • strawberry tongue

17.19.) <u>RESPIRATORY TRACT INFECTIONS</u>

		CAUSED BY:
croup	• usually viral • **gradual onset** • low fever o *stridor improves with epinephrine*	**parainfluenza virus**
epiglottitis [1]	• **acute onset** • high fever • "thumb-print sign" on x-ray o *some relief with neck extension ("sniffing dog position")*	*haemophilus influenzae*
tracheitis	• **gradual onset** • high fever • subglottal narrowing	**bacterial** (*Staph. aureus*)
bronchiolitis	• children 2 to 6 months • variable fever • respiratory distress • rhonchi, wheezes, rales o *does not respond to bronchodilators*	**viral** (RSV)

Hospitalize immediately and do not examine with tongue blade unless ready to intubate because of the risk of triggering a fatal airway obstruction.

17.20.) <u>RHEUMATIC FEVER</u>

Rheumatic fever occurs mostly in school age children with untreated streptococcal pharyngitis. Rheumatic heart disease is a feared sequelae and occurs many years after rheumatic fever.

major criteria	<ul><li>carditis</li><li>polyarthritis</li><li>chorea</li><li>erythema marginatum</li><li>subcutaneous nodules</li></ul>
minor criteria	<ul><li>○ fever</li><li>○ arthralgia</li><li>○ elevated acute phase reactants</li></ul>

- **ASO titer** performed to confirm <u>past</u> infection with Group A β-hemolytic streptococci

- **rapid antigen assay** if suspected acute infection.
- if negative result and still suspected: throat swab and culture.

- Penicillin within 10 days of infection prevents rheumatic fever.

17.21.) CHILDHOOD TUMORS

Leukemias are the most common malignancies affecting children. Brain tumors are the most common solid malignancies and neuroblastoma is the most common extracranial tumor of children. Prognosis is significantly better than in adults!

brain tumors	• infratentorial more common than supratentorial • astrocytoma more common than medulloblastoma • MRI is study of choice • no lumbar puncture (risk of herniation!)
neuroblastoma	• **typical age: 2 years** • **typical** presentation : asymptomatic abdominal mass • arises from neural crest *(displaces urinary collecting system)* o survival about 80% in young children *(poorer in older children)*
Wilms' tumor	• **typical age: 2-5 years** • **typical presentation : asymptomatic abdominal mass** • arises anywhere within kidney *(distorts urinary collecting system)* o survival about 85%
Ewing's sarcoma	• **typical age : 10-15 years** • severe limb pain (causing awakening at night) • arises from medullary cavity (commonly : femur) o survival < 40%
histiocytosis	• **typical age : infants, young children** • typical presentation: fever, weight loss, anemia • multiple disease entities • lytic bone lesions o may resolve spontaneously or require chemotherapy

17.22.) <u>CHILD ABUSE</u>

It is difficult to determine whether injuries in a child are accidental or intentional. Here are some clues:

PERHAPS ACCIDENTAL	PROBABLY INTENTIONAL
• splash marks • injuries to front • foot soles spared	• clearly demarcated areas, no splash • injuries to back • foot soles involved o history of multiple injuries o retinal hemorrhage (shaken baby)

 *As physician **you are not supposed to play detective.** If you suspect abuse, report it to the Department of Social Services.*

> ### <u>FORMS OF ABUSE:</u>
> (1.) physical
> (2.) emotional
> (3.) sexual
> (4.) neglect

MEASLES
➢ Supportive only
➢ Avoid salicylates (better: acetaminophen)
➢ Immunoglobulin effective if given within first 6 days

MUMPS
➢ Supportive only
➢ Orchitis: analgesics and scrotal support
➢ Unilateral nerve deafness: usually transient

RUBELLA
➢ Teratogenic (especially during first trimester)
➢ Seropositive mothers are immune
➢ Seroconversion in first trimester indicates high risk: consider abortion

CHICKEN POX
➢ Supportive measures, trim nails so infant's can't scratch
➢ Diphenhydramine for itching
➢ Prevent secondary bacterial infections
➢ Acyclovir (topical or systemic) for ocular infection

PERTUSSIS
➢ Erythromycin for patient and household contacts
   (regardless of age or immunization status)
➢ Nutritional support: frequent small feedings (if necessary: parental fluid)
➢ Cough suppressants are of little benefit

MENINGITIS
➤ Lumbar puncture and blood culture if any suspicion
➤ Empiric treatment: cefotaxime (plus ampicillin)
➤ If seizures develop: suspect encephalitis

HIV POSITIVE CHILD
➤ HIV antibody test is unreliable in children < 6 months
➤ Vaccinate at usual intervals, but give inactivated polio rather than oral
➤ Combination therapy: AZT + non-nucleotide inhibitors + protease inhibitors
➤ PCP prophylaxis: recommended for all infants with HIV, regardless of CD4 count!

RESPIRATORY DISTRESS SYNDROME
➤ Oxygen supplementation
(Intubate and ventilate if in respiratory failure - PEEP)
➤ Corticosteroids and cromolyn to decrease inflammation and risk of bronchopulmonary dysplasia
➤ Intratracheal application of artificial surfactant

SUDDEN INFANT DEATH SYNDROME
supine versus prone sleeping position:
➤ Preterm infants with respiratory distress or infants with gastroesophageal reflux do better sleeping in prone position
➤ Positioning infant on their side or back (supine) reduces risk for SIDS

CYSTIC FIBROSIS
➤ Prognosis usually limited by lung disease
➤ Common infections: initially *Staph. aureus*, later *Pseudomonas*
➤ Chest physiotherapy, antibiotics, bronchodilators...

ASD

- Determine pulmonary vs. systemic blood flow (cardiac catheter oximetry)
- If > 2:1 consider surgical correction (best done at ages 2-4 years)
- If untreated: shunt reversal and heart failure common in third and fourth decade.

VSD

- If small expect spontaneous closure
- Elective surgery at 2-4 years
- Significant pulmonary hypertension is a contraindication for surgery!

PDA

- Try indomethacin to facilitate spontaneous closure
- Elective surgery at 1-2 years
- Operate early if large left to right shunt persists

FALLOT'S TETRALOGY

- Consider palliative surgery for very small severely cyanotic infants
  (create Gore-Tex shunt between subclavian and pulmonary artery)
- Total correction: between birth and age 2 years
  (surgical mortality up to 5%)

TRANSPOSITION OF THE GREAT VESSELS

- Newborn: palliative enlargement of atrial septal defect
  ("pull-through" of balloon catheter)
- Anatomic correction at 6 months (high surgical mortality)

TRACHEOESOPHAGEAL FISTULA
- Elevate head of bed to prevent esophageal reflux into lung
- Drainage of blind pouch
- Surgical correction
- Evaluate for other abnormalities

PYLORIC STENOSIS
- Pyloromyotomy

INTUSSUSCEPTION
- Fatal if untreated
- Barium enema is diagnostic and therapeutic
  (surgery if unsuccessful or perforation)

MECONIUM ILEUS OR PLUG
- Suspect cystic fibrosis!
- Contrast enema may be therapeutic in case of plug
- Get rectal biopsy if you suspect Hirschsprung's disease

MALROTATION OF SMALL INTESTINE
- High risk of ischemia, necrosis, perforation and sepsis
- Surgical repair

HIRSCHSPRUNG'S DISEASE
- Surgery: Initially: temporary colostomy or ileostomy
            At 6 months of age: resection of aganglionic segment

INFANTILE BOTULISM
- Prevention: avoid contaminated food (honey!)
- Antitoxin neutralizes circulating but not (irreversibly) bound toxin
- Bed rest, fluids
- Ventilation if necessary

CRYPTORCHISM

(if uncorrected: failure of spermatogenesis, increased risk for malignancy, but normal androgen production)

If present at birth:
➤ Observe: 80% of undescended testes are in the scrotum by age of 1 year
➤ Surgical repair (orchiopexy) should be performed at age of 1 years
➤ If bilateral: rule out that patient isn't a fully virilized female

If detected at puberty:
➤ Testis should be removed because of cancer risk

POLYCYSTIC KIDNEYS

➤ Diagnosis: ultrasound
➤ Monitor renal function
➤ Manage complications of renal failure
➤ Strict blood pressure control
➤ Genetic counseling

WILM'S TUMOR

➤ Resection plus multi-agent adjuvant chemotherapy
➤ Cure rates up to 90%

HENOCH SCHÖNLEIN PURPURA

➤ Usually self limited: supportive care only
➤ Corticosteroids if gastrointestinal hemorrhage is present

CONGENITAL ADRENAL HYPERPLASIA
> Goal: suppression of endogenous ACTH

Lifelong daily oral hydrocortisone:
> Increase dose 3 to 5fold during periods of stress (fever, surgery etc.)

Lifelong daily mineralocorticoid if salt wasting:
> Does not need to be adjusted for stress

CONGENITAL HYPOTHYROIDISM
> Primary prevention: iodine supplementation prevents endemic hypothyroidism (cretinism)
> Secondary prevention: mandatory screening programs (T4, TSH)
> Levothyroxine for maintenance therapy

WILSON'S DISEASE
(hepatolenticular degeneration)
> Lifelong penicillamine for symptomatic and asymptomatic cases
> Dietary copper restriction not practical
> Daily vit. B6 to prevent optical neuritis

CEREBRAL PALSY

- ➢ Prevention: improved prenatal care and obstetric management
- ➢ Physical, occupational and speech therapy
- ➢ Spasticity can sometimes be reduced with diazepam or baclofen

POLIOMYELITIS

- ➢ Most cases in the US occur in immunodeficient patients who received live vaccine
- ➢ Bed rest, fever and pain control
- ➢ Intubation and assisted ventilation may be necessary

FEBRILE SEIZURES

- ➢ Anticonvulsants (phenobarbital) only for high risk infants with recurrent febrile seizures
- ➢ If age of onset < 1 year or duration > 15 min: increased likelihood of future chronic epileptic disorder

REYE'S SYNDROME

(encephalopathy with acute fatty liver degeneration)
- ➢ Nasogastric tube, Foley catheter
- ➢ Ventilation may become necessary
- ➢ Treat increased intracranial pressure: - hyperventilation
  - mannitol infusions,
  - ventricular drainage
- ➢ Vitamin K, intramuscular

RETINOBLASTOMA

(white pupil reflex)
- ➢ Enucleation, radiotherapy. Goal: minimize tumor, maximize vision
- ➢ Adjuvant chemotherapy if optic nerve is involved

INJURY
AND
POISONING

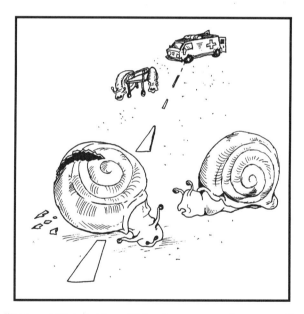

"Easy, John, help will be here any day now."

18.1.) HEAD TRAUMA

	SIGNS & SYMPTOMS
concussion	CT: normal • brief loss of consciousness • no identifiable neuropathological changes • transient amnesia (anterograde and retrograde)
contusion	• cerebral edema • diffuse intracerebral hemorrhage (coup and contra-coup) if **localized:** focal signs if **generalized:** focal signs plus impaired mentation
epidural hematoma	CT: lenticular shape (convex) • injury of arteries (often middle meningeal artery) • brief lucid interval, followed by headache and rapidly decreasing level of consciousness
subdural hematoma	CT: follows outline of skull (concave) • injury of bridging veins • often delayed for days or weeks after injury • more common in elderly and alcoholics

basilar skull fractures	• often missed on x-ray
	
	• watch for signs: - hemotympanum
	                        - mastoid ecchymosis
	                        - periorbital ecchymosis
	                        - facial palsy
	                        - CSF in nasal sinuses

18.2.) <u>CHEST TRAUMA</u>

	SIGNS & SYMPTOMS
pneumothorax	• spontaneous or following trauma • sudden chest pain • hyperresonance
tension pneumothorax	• sudden chest pain, hyperresonance • ventilatory and circulatory compromise • mediastinal shift • rapidly fatal
open pneumothorax	• from penetrating injury • small wounds may create tension pneumothorax (valvelike mechanism)
hemothorax	• penetrating or blunt trauma • often combined with pneumothorax • shock, hypotension
flail chest	• multiple rib fractures • unstable segment moves inward during inspiration ("paradoxical movement") • respiratory distress
pulmonary contusion	• a/w rib fractures • pulmonary infiltrates on CXR • hypoxemia
cardiac tamponade	• penetrating chest trauma • hypotension • jugular vein distention (unless patient is severely hypovolemic)
aortic dissection	• often fatal • progressive hypotension and shock • mediastinal widening

18.3.) <u>ABDOMINAL TRAUMA</u>

	SIGNS & SYMPTOMS
hemorrhage	• injury of: liver, spleen, vessels *if shock and hypotension are present: assume intra-abdominal hemorrhage until excluded by CT, laparoscopy or lavage*
peritonitis	• intestinal injury • pancreatic injury • fever, tachycardia, diffuse pain, ileus
spleen rupture	**most common injury of blunt abdominal trauma** • left upper quadrant pain • may radiate to shoulder • intra-abdominal hemorrhage (shock, hypotension, peritoneal signs) • CT scan is highly sensitive
liver injury	**most common injury of penetrating abdominal trauma** • right upper quadrant pain • intra-abdominal hemorrhage (shock, hypotension, peritoneal signs)
intestinal injury	• usually due to penetrating trauma • small intestinal injury is more common • large intestinal injury is more severe (peritonitis)

<u>INDICATIONS FOR PERITONEAL LAVAGE:</u>
(1.) unexplained hypotension and shock
(2.) low thoracic penetrating wounds
(3.) inability to evaluate abdomen (spinal cord trauma, unconscious patient)

18.4.) <u>ACUTE ABDOMEN</u>

Acute abdomen is a sudden, non-traumatic condition that may require urgent surgery: pain, abdominal rigidity and signs of shock are typical.

	CONSIDER:
female patient ?	<ul><li>ruptured ectopic pregnancy</li><li>ruptured ovarian cyst</li><li>torsion of ovarian tumor</li></ul>
evidence of trauma ?	<ul><li>perforation</li><li>hemorrhage</li></ul>
evidence of obstruction ?	<ul><li>intussusception</li><li>volvulus</li><li>incarcerated hernia</li></ul>
evidence of peritonitis ?	<ul><li>appendicitis</li><li>diverticulitis</li><li>pancreatitis</li></ul>
hypovolemic shock ?	<ul><li>ruptured aortic aneurysm</li></ul>
others	<ul><li>toxins</li><li>gastroenteritis</li><li>UTI</li></ul>

18.5.) <u>GENITOURINARY TRAUMA</u>

	SIGNS & SYMPTOMS
bladder rupture	• common with pelvic fractures • **gross hematuria** (urine sample by catheterization) • acute abdomen indicates intraperitoneal rupture
urethra disruption	• **high prostate** on rectal exam • bloody urethral discharge • may result in impotence and incontinence
kidneys	• common in motor vehicle accidents • degree of hematuria not related to degree of injury • flank pain, lower rib fractures <u>Minor injury</u>: • subcapsular hematomas • contusions <u>Major injury</u>: • vascular injury • deep lacerations • retroperitoneal hemorrhage

18.6.) <u>FRACTURES</u>

hip	<ul><li>osteoporosis</li><li>**risk of avascular necrosis of femur head**</li></ul>
ribs	<ul><li>**pain that worsens with deep breathing**</li><li>flail chest: inward movement during inspiration</li></ul>
Colle's	<ul><li>breakage and displacement of distal radius</li><li>**from fall on outstretched hand**</li></ul>
elbow	<ul><li>more common in children</li><li>watch for injury of median nerve and radial artery</li><li>**avoid Volkmann's contracture** (ischemic damage)</li></ul>
pelvis	<ul><li>most commonly due to motor vehicle accident</li><li>**blood loss!**</li></ul>
tibia	<ul><li><u>Compartment syndrome:</u> pain, pulseless, puffy, paresthesia, paralysis</li></ul>
Pott's	<ul><li>fracture of distal fibula and torn off internal malleolus</li><li>**following foot eversion and abduction**</li></ul>

 Avascular necrosis most common of - femur head
- navicular wrist bone

18.7.) <u>NERVE INJURIES</u>

DAMAGE TO :	RESULTS IN IMPAIRED FUNCTION OF :
axillary nerve	shoulder abduction
long thoracic nerve	serratus anterior muscle ("winged scapula")
musculocutaneous nerve	elbow flexion
median nerve	thumb extension
ulnar nerve	index finger abduction
femoral nerve	knee extension
obturator nerve	hip adduction
superior gluteal nerve	hip abduction
inferior gluteal nerve	hip extension
tibial nerve	foot plantar flexion
peroneal nerve	foot eversion

18.8.) DROWNING

A) DROWNING:

drowning	• death from fluid aspiration (90%) • or due to laryngospasm (10%) • freshwater (hypotonic) may cause intravascular hemolysis (otherwise little difference to sea water drowning)
near-drowning	**Monitor patient for:** • pulmonary edema • pneumonitis • adult respiratory distress syndrome • cerebral edema • cardiac arrhythmias

B) DIVING:

decompression sickness (Caisson disease)	• rapid ascent from deep sea diving • rapid ascent in unpressurized aircraft • symptoms occur **within 30 min to hours** o joint pain o skin mottling o burning, prickling sensation o cough, dyspnea o coma
arterial gas embolism	• rapid ascent from deep diving • symptoms occur **within minutes** o seizures o myocardial infarction

18.9.) <u>HIGH ALTITUDE SICKNESS</u>

symptoms	• headache, dizziness • nausea, vomiting
feared complications	**<u>Pulmonary edema:</u>** • severe dyspnea at rest, orthopnea and wheezing **<u>Cerebral edema:</u>** • ataxia, confusion • papilledema, retinal hemorrhage

18.10.) <u>ANTIDOTES</u>

INTOXICATION	ANTIDOTE
acetaminophen	N-acetylcysteine
opiates	naloxone
benzodiazepines	flumazenil
opioids	naloxone
methanol, ethylene glycol	ethanol
CO	100% O_2
cyanide	amyl nitrate
organophosphates	atropine, pralidoxime
iron	deferoxamine
lead	EDTA
coumarin	Vit. K
heparin	protamine

 Intoxication with acidic drugs (e.g. barbiturate, salicylate): *Alkalinize urine (IV sodium-bicarbonate) to enhance renal excretion.*

HEAD TRAUMA
➢ **Concussion:** careful observation
➢ **Epidural hematoma:** urgent surgery to avoid brain herniation
➢ **Acute subdural hematoma:** surgery
➢ **Slow subdural hematoma:** this is the "classic" high risk patient who becomes symptomatic days or weeks after the incident

CHEST TRAUMA
➢ **Rib fractures:** analgesia, encourage patient to cough and breathe!
➢ **Flail chest:** may require endotracheal intubation, monitor blood gases
➢ **Pneumothorax:** convert tension pneumothorax to open pneumothorax
➢ **Great vessel injury:** emergency thoracostomy

ABDOMINAL TRAUMA
➢ **Penetrating gun shot wounds:** surgery
➢ **Splenic rupture:** splenectomy or repair if possible
                              (urgent if patient has falling hematocrit or blood pressure)

PELVIC TRAUMA
➢ Monitor patient for hemorrhagic shock
➢ Urethral bleeding: obtain urethrogram before inserting a Foley catheter
   (Microhematuria found by catheter but no shock or pelvic fracture: observe)
➢ Bladder rupture: repair, unless small and extraperitoneal

SPRAINS
➢ Rest, ice, compression, elevation
➢ NSAIDs
➢ Knee joint: early mobilization important

DISLOCATIONS
- Morphine to reduce pain and allow muscle relaxation
- Immediate closed reduction
- Shoulder dislocation: anterior is easier to fix than posterior dislocation

HIP DISLOCATION
(usually posterior, often due to motor vehicle accidents)
- Urgent reduction (usually "open") required to avoid avascular necrosis of femur head

FRACTURES
- **Clavicle:** posterior T-splint
- **Humerus:** hanging cast, exercise to prevent stiffening of shoulder. If fracture is distal watch out for Volkmann's ischemic contracture!
- **Radius, ulna:** closed (or open) reduction, intraosseus pins
- **Wrist:** scaphoid fractures are easily overlooked and are a common site of non-union
- **Cervical vertebrae:** if suspected: immobilize immediately
- **Pelvis:** 6-8 weeks bed rest
- **Femur neck:** (common site of non-union) → internal fixation.
  (avoid abduction plaster cast)
- **Tibia (±fibula):** plaster splint
- **Pott's:** closed reduction, plaster cast

DROWNING
- "The patient isn't dead until he/she is warm and dead"
  (immersion in cold water slows brain metabolism to an amazing extent)
- Resuscitate immediately
  (don't waste time attempting to drain water from victims lungs or stomach)
- If patient survives: hospitalize and watch for signs of pneumonitis or pulmonary edema

DECOMPRESSION SICKNESS

- Oxygen
- Analgesics
- Consider recompression

BURNS

- Rule of 9*: head 1, arms 1+1, legs 2+2, front torso 2, back torso 2
- Large volume fluid resuscitation (crystalloids).
  (Adjust to maintain urine output > 0.5 ml/kg/h)
- Expect cardiac arrhythmias due to electrolyte imbalances
- Expect ileus if > 20% surface burned

11 areas that count for 9% each

POISONING

- Gastric lavage is better than inducing vomiting
- Do not induce vomiting if patient unconscious
- Do not induce vomiting if caustics or hydrocarbons (oils) have been ingested

- Give 50-100 g activated charcoal (except for acetaminophen overdose)
- Specific antidotes see (18.10)

INSECT STINGS

Anaphylaxis (rapid onset of urticaria, respiratory distress and hypotension):
- ➤ Antihistamines
- ➤ Epinephrine
- ➤ May require intubation

ANIMAL BITES

- ➤ Risk of infection: monkey > cat > dog bites
- ➤ Cleanse, debride and irrigate wound
- ➤ Cephalosporins for cat and dog bites
- ➤ Hospitalize if infection involves hand
- ➤ Consider rabies prophylaxis
  (duck embryo vaccine plus hyperimmune rabies immune globulins (HRIG) obtained from human volunteers)

SPIDER BITES

- ➤ Black widow spider[1]:   - Ca-gluconate
- ➤ Brown recluse spider[2]: - glucocorticoids
                             - may require total excision of lesion

---

[1] *abdominal pain, vomiting, shock*
[2] *fever, rash, jaundice, DIC*

 In the unlikely event that a skunk or bat bites you, the doctor recommends rabies prophylaxis!

NEUROLOGY

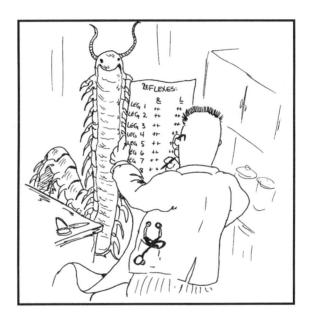

19.1.) <u>CEREBROSPINAL FLUID</u>

Do not delay antibiotic treatment to wait for results of lumbar puncture when suspecting bacterial meningitis!

CSF CHANGES IN MENINGITIS:

	BACTERIAL	TB	FUNGAL	VIRAL
cells	PMNs	lymphocytes	lymphocytes	lymphocytes
glucose [1]	↓	(↓)	(↓)	∅
protein	↑	(↑)	(↑)	∅

[1] *normal is about 2/3 of serum glucose value.*

<u>INDICATIONS FOR LUMBAR PUNCTURE:</u>
(1.) suspicion of acute CNS infection
(2.) before anticoagulant therapy of stroke if imaging unavailable

<u>CONTRAINDICATIONS FOR LUMBAR PUNCTURE:</u>
(1.) suspicion of brain tumor
(2.) increased intracranial pressure (check retina for papilledema!)
(3.) bleeding tendency

 CSF of newborns: *higher protein content, more lymphocytes.*

308

19.2.) <u>PUPILS</u>

The pupillary light reflex is such an important diagnostic tool because it involves nuclei near the vital brainstem centers:

Optic nerve → Edinger Westphal nucleus → Oculomotor nerve

	LIGHT REACTIVE	NOT LIGHT REACTIVE
large	• children • anxiety	• death • atropine poisoning • cocaine, amphetamine
small	• elderly • Horner's syndrome	• Argyll-Robertson • opiates

Argyll-Robertson pupils constrict to near accommodation but do not respond to light.

19.3.) HEADACHE

tension headache	• **steady, non-pulsating** • unilateral or bilateral
classic migraine	• **preceded by aura** • malaise • nausea • photophobia
common migraine	• **not preceded by aura** • malaise • nausea • photophobia
complicated migraine	• **migraine with neurologic symptoms that outlast the headache (ischemia):** - paresthesias - aphasia
cluster headache	• **severe, unilateral, orbital pain** • occurs in clusters lasting weeks • conjunctiva injection • eyelid edema • lacrimation
tumor headache	• **develops slowly with increased intracranial pressure** • initially mild, occurs after waking up • exacerbated by coughing, bending or sudden movements
meningitis	• **severe throbbing pain**
subarachnoid hemorrhage	• sudden onset headache • **"worst ever"**

19.4.) VERTIGO

Vertigo is a sensation of rotational movement and patients may lose their balance, risking injury. It is due to diseases of the inner ear, vestibulocochlear nerve or cerebellum.

physiologic vertigo	• **mismatch between vestibular, visual and somatosensory input** o motion sickness o height vertigo o astronauts
brainstem ischemia / tumors	• **vertigo** • **diplopia** • **nausea, vomiting** o occipital headaches
Ménière's	• **abrupt, severe vertigo** • **fluctuating hearing loss** • **tinnitus** o usually unilateral
labyrinthitis	• **abrupt, severe vertigo** o patient unable to sit or stand o nystagmus: away from involved labyrinth

<u>Other causes of "dizziness" that might be confused with vertigo:</u>
(1.) ataxia (cerebellar disease or loss of proprioception)
(2.) syncope
(3.) anxiety
(4.) partial complex seizures

19.5.) <u>SYNCOPE</u>

Transient losses of consciousness can be due to cardiovascular or neurological problems.

A) <u>CARDIOVASCULAR</u>:

	ADDITIONAL SYMPTOMS:
vasovagal	• due to stress or pain • preceded by nausea, pallor, sweating
cardiac	**tachyarrhythmias:** • preceded by dizziness, palpitations **outflow obstruction:** (cardiomyopathy, aortic stenosis etc.) • precipitated by exertion

B) <u>NEUROLOGICAL</u>:

	ADDITIONAL SYMPTOMS:
TIA	• transient focal signs
seizures	• aura • tongue biting • incontinence • postictal confusion
hypoglycemia	• preceded by confusion, jitteriness, tachycardia

 "Coma-Cocktail": *give thiamine, glucose, naloxone.*

19.6.) <u>STROKE</u>

It is most important to distinguish between hemorrhagic and ischemic stroke to make treatment decisions (CT or MRI).

TIA	• <u>transient</u> focal neurologic deficits • lasts minutes to hours • no residual effect
ischemic	• **embolic or thrombotic occlusion** Risk factors: • arteriosclerosis • atrial fibrillation • heart valves (septic or non-septic)
hemorrhagic	• **subarachnoid or intracerebral** Risk factors: • intracranial aneurysms • arteriovenous malformations • hypertension
middle cerebral artery	• contralateral hemiparesis • aphasia
anterior cerebral artery	• contralateral foot and distal leg paresis
vertebral and basilar artery	• amnesia, diplopia, ataxia • visual field defects
lacunar stroke (small branches of Willis' circle)	**pure motor hemiparesis:** internal capsule **pure sensory stroke:** ventrolateral thalamus **dysarthria, clumsy hand:** base of pons

A young woman with stroke: think 1.) oral contraceptives
2.) SLE

19.7.) <u>CORTICAL SIGNS</u>

Important signs of cortical damage (stroke, tumors, degeneration):

FRONTAL LOBE	PARIETAL LOBE
• contralateral UMN lesion (spastic paresis) • personality changes	• contralateral impairment of somatesthetic recognition • spatial disorientation • inappropriate affect
<u>If dominant hemisphere:</u> • aphasia	<u>If dominant hemisphere:</u> • aphasia • apraxia • acalculia

19.8.) <u>APHASIA</u>

Broca's	• **inferior frontal gyrus** o nonfluent speech o good comprehension o self aware, frustrated patient
Wernicke's	• **posterior superior temporal lobe** o fluent but nonsensical speech o poor comprehension o often no insight
global	• **large frontal-temporal lesions** o defects in both expression and comprehension

Don't confuse Broca's aphasia with dysarthria (inability to articulate properly due to a motor disorder).

19.9.) TREMOR

The basal ganglia and cerebellum modulate the motor output of the cortico-spinal tract and if damaged can cause tremors (oscillations) or dyskinesias (involuntary non-repetitive patterns). The quality of the tremor gives important clues to diagnosis:

physiological	• 8 to 12 Hz • distal extremities
Parkinson's	• 4 to 7 Hz • **resting tremor** • "pill rolling"
cerebellar	• 3 to 6 Hz • **intention tremor** • increases when target is approached
asterixis	• 1 to 3 Hz • **wrist joint flapping**

19.10.) <u>EPILEPSY</u>

generalized seizures (involves both hemispheres)	**nonconvulsive** • absence spells (petit mal) 1 • myoclonic seizures **convulsive** • tonic-clonic (grand mal)

partial seizures	**simple**
	(normal consciousness)
	• motor (Jacksonian)
	• sensory (auditory, olfactory...)
	• autonomic (pallor, flushing...)
	
	complex [2]
	(impaired consciousness)
	• most frequent form of chronic epilepsy
	
	• origin in temporal lobe or limbic area
	
	   aura: - déja vu
	            - foul odor
	            - pleasure, fear, anger
	            - lip smacking

[1] *no aura, no warning, no cataplexy, no postictal period.*
[2] *most frequent form of chronic epilepsy*

 Partial seizures often progress to secondarily generalized seizures.

Narcolepsy = REM onset sleep:
(1.) involuntary daytime sleep
(2.) cataplexy
(3.) hypnagogic hallucinations

19.11.) <u>EEG PATTERNS</u>

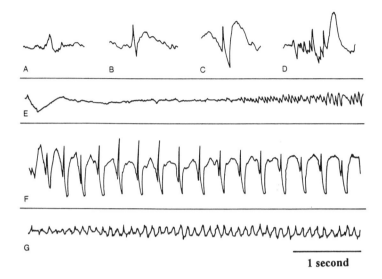

From *Cecil Textbook of Medicine*, 19th edition, p. 2208, edited by J.B. Wyngaarden et al. Copyright 1992 by W.B. Saunders Co., Philadelphia, PA. Used with permission.

A:	interictal sharp wave
B:	interictal spike-and-wave complex
C:	interictal spike-and-wave complex
D:	interictal polyspike-and-wave complex
E:	onset of generalized convulsion
F:	3/sec spike-and-wave complex (petit mal)
G:	temporal lobe seizure

19.12.) <u>BACTERIAL MENINGITIS</u>

neonates (< 1 month)	1. E. coli 2. **Streptococcus agalactia** 3. Listeria
children (1 month ~ 15 years)	1. **Meningococcus** 2. Pneumococcus
adults (>15 years)	1. **Pneumococcus** 2. Meningococcus

<u>Initial treatment</u> is empiric, based on the most likely organisms:

Pneumococcus	➢ penicillin ➢ ampicillin ➢ ceftriaxone
Meningococcus	➢ same as for pneumococcus <u>Prophylaxis:</u> ➢ rifampin ➢ tetravalent vaccine (ages >2 years)
Listeria	➢ penicillin ➢ ampicillin
Haemophilus [1]	➢ cefotaxime

[1] *has become rare due to vaccination!*

 Viral meningitis: *Enteroviruses > Arboviruses (Summer!), Herpes*

19.13.) <u>MOTOR NEURON LESIONS</u>

Distinguish lesions to the "upper motor neuron" (corticospinal tract) and lesions
to the "lower motor neuron" (α-motoneuron from spinal cord to muscle):

UPPER MOTOR NEURON	LOWER MOTOR NEURON
• spastic paralysis	• flaccid paralysis • fibrillations • fasciculations • atrophy
• increased tendon reflexes • Babinski reflex present	• reflexes decreased or absent

---

FIBRILLATIONS:
(1.) spontaneous twitching of single denervated
    muscle fibers due to ACH hypersensitivity
(2.) can not be seen through skin

FASCICULATIONS:
(1.) spontaneous twitching of motor units
(2.) can be seen through skin

19.14.) <u>SPINAL CORD SIGNS</u>

To understand the characteristic patterns of spinal cord injury, you should review the major pathways (1.) corticospinal tract, (2.) dorsal columns and (3.) spinothalamic tract.

Brown-Séquard (trauma, tumors)	<u>ipsilateral</u>: • spastic hemiparesis • loss of position and vibration <u>contralateral</u>: • loss of pain and temperature
anterior cord (occlusion of anterior spinal artery)	• **spastic paresis** • **loss of pain and temperature** o intact position and vibration
posterolateral cord (syphilis, MS)	• **ataxia** • **loss of position and vibration** o intact pain and temperature
syringomyelia (often congenital)	<u>lower neck, shoulders, arms, hands</u>: • loss of pain and temperature • wasting of muscles o intact pain and temperature
Guillain-Barré (acute postinfectious polyneuropathy)	• **motor paralysis:** bilateral, ascending, flaccid • **sensory deficit**

19.15.) PERIPHERAL NEUROPATHIES

Peripheral neuropathies are often characterized by a "sock-glove pattern" of sensory and motor deficits, but can also affect specific subsets of neurons (for example motor neurons in ALS). Nerve conduction velocity tests can help to confirm the diagnosis, but not the etiology:

	TYPICAL CAUSES
hereditary	• Charcot-Marie-Tooth • Friedreich's ataxia • leukodystrophies
toxins	• lead • arsenic • mercury • many drugs
nutritional	• Vit. B6 deficiency • Vit. B12 deficiency • Vit. E deficiency
other acquired	• Guillain-Barré syndrome • amyotrophic lateral sclerosis • diabetes mellitus

---

CHARCOT JOINT:
caused by loss of proprioception (tabes, diabetic neuropathy...)
→ repeat trauma
→ joint instability, painless swelling

19.16.) <u>SLEEP DISORDERS</u>

In patients with insomnia you first must exclude specific causes such as emotional problems, chronic pain, alcohol or drug abuse. Sleep apnea is surprisingly common and an important cause of daytime sleepiness.

insomnia	• difficulty initiating sleep • difficulty maintaining sleep ○ exclude medical conditions ○ exclude mental disorders such as anxiety or major depressive disorder
sleep apnea	• **obstructive** a/w obesity (common!) • **central** brain stem disorder (rare!)
daytime hypersomnia	• prolonged sleep • daytime sleep ○ often the result of insomnia or sleep apnea
narcolepsy	• REM onset sleep **cataplexy:** sudden loss of muscle tone **hypnagogic hallucinations:** at sleep onset **hypnopompic hallucinations:** at awakening **sleep paralysis:** upon awakening

<u>PROMOTE SLEEP HYGIENE:</u>
(1.) Regular sleep time and regular bed time routine
(2.) Don't use bedroom for activities other than sleep (and sex)
(3.) Don't eat or exercise before going to bed

TENSION HEADACHE

- ➤ Mild analgesics: acetaminophen, aspirin, ibuprofen...
- ➤ If chronic and severe: add antidepressant
- ➤ Teach relaxation techniques

MIGRAINE AND CLUSTER HEADACHE

Acute attack:
- ➤ Sumatriptan (serotonin agonist)
- ➤ Ergotamine plus caffeine

Prophylaxis:
- ➤ If > 2 attacks per month: β-blockers, calcium antagonists...

TRIGEMINAL NEURALGIA

- ➤ Carbamazepine provides relief most cases
- ➤ If refractory: add baclofen

TIA

- ➤ Get MRI or CT scan to exclude hemorrhage
- ➤ Anticoagulation
- ➤ Carotid endarterectomy if stenosis > 70% and relatively little atherosclerosis elsewhere in the cerebrovascular circulation

STROKE

- ➤ Get MRI or CT scan to distinguish ischemia from hemorrhage

Ischemic stroke:
- ➤ Tissue plasminogen activator within first 3 hours (unless risk of hemorrhage!)
- ➤ Anticoagulation: IV heparin, then warfarin
- ➤ Corticosteroids may help to reduce cerebral edema

Hemorrhage:
- ➤ Bed rest, avoid straining
- ➤ Non-opiate pain relief
- ➤ Aneurysm → surgical clipping as soon as possible to prevent rebleeding
- ➤ Prognosis is poor compared to ischemic stroke

GRAND MAL

➤ Many patients have a single seizure with no recurrence: after a first attack, long-term treatment is only indicated if a cause can be found.
➤ Monitor drug levels regularly
➤ Never abruptly discontinue anticonvulsants

STATUS EPILEPTICUS

➤ Assure airways, obtain IV access
➤ Glucose infusion
➤ Diazepam IV
➤ If convulsions persist → increase dose or add phenobarbital
➤ If convulsions still persist → anesthesia, neuromuscular blockade

ABSENCE SEIZURES (PETIT MAL)

➤ Half of children with petit mal will develop clonic-tonic seizures before age 20
➤ Ethosuximide

NARCOLEPSY

(Avoid heavy meals, especially before the USMLE exam)
➤ Methylphenidate (Ritalin) or other amphetamine-like stimulant

SLEEP APNEA

➤ Sleep study to distinguish obstructive from central apnea
➤ **Obstructive:** - weight reduction
             - continuous positive airway pressure at night
             - for severe cases: remove tonsils, adenoid, uvula
➤ **Central:** protriptyline

PARKINSON'S
- **Early stage:** anticholinergics, amantadine
- **Advanced:** gradually increasing carbidopa/levodopa as tolerated (dyskinesias)
- **Late stage:** when response to levodopa diminishes ("on/off" phenomenon) add anticholinergics or bromocriptine

ALZHEIMER'S
- Search for and correct treatable factors contributing to cognitive impairment (depression, endocrine disturbances, multi-drug use, nutritional deficiencies...)
- Enhance cholinergic neurotransmission: donepezil or tacrine
- *Gingko biloba* extract may improve memory
- Advance directive should be drafted as early as possible

HUNTINGTON'S
- Phenothiazines or haloperidol to suppress dyskinesias
- Reserpine to deplete central monoamine stores may be useful
- Offer genetic counseling: (1/2 of patient's children are at risk!)

MULTIPLE SCLEROSIS
- Glucocorticoids hasten recovery from <u>acute</u> relapse (but do not use for long-term treatment)
- β-interferon appears to reduce relapse rate
- Consider immunosuppressive therapy for rapidly progressive active MS
- Baclofen or dantrolene to improve spasticity

GUILLAIN-BARRÉ SYNDROME
- Medical emergency! Monitor and support vital function!
- <u>Early</u> plasmapheresis or IV immune globulin improves outcome
- Corticosteroids are not indicated (will delay recovery!)
- Many patients have residual weakness even after years...

PSYCHIATRY

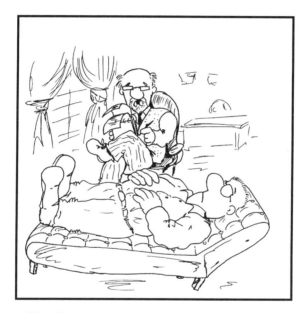

"And how long have you been, in my opinion, evil?"

20.1.) GENETIC FACTORS

No single gene <u>causing</u> major psychoses has been identified. Nevertheless, twin studies suggest a strong genetic component to schizophrenia and bipolar disorder and it is assumed that these somehow render the patient vulnerable to particular life experiences.

schizophrenia	• **50% monozygotic twin concordance** • 12% if one parent has disorder • 40% if both parents have disorder
major depressive disorder	• **50% monozygotic twin concordance** • genetic component not as strong as for bipolar I disorder
bipolar I disorder	• **50-90% monozygotic twin concordance** • 25% if one parent has disorder • 50% if both parents have disorder
mental retardation	**cause often unknown** the more severe the mental retardation, the more likely it is due to infections, toxins or trauma (often perinatal) **<u>chromosomal abnormalities</u>:** • Fragile X • Prader-Willi • Cri-du-chat • Down syndrome

20.2.) <u>DSM IV CLASSIFICATION</u>

A complete psychiatric diagnosis should contain 5 elements or "axes":

Axis I	- **psychiatric** diagnosis [1]
Axis II	- **personality** disorders - mental retardation
Axis III	- **general medical** conditions
Axis IV	- **social** and environmental problems
Axis V	- level of functioning

[1] *psychiatric diagnosis except mental retardation or personality disorders, which should be coded on axis II.*

DSM IV © 1994 American Psychiatric Association. Definitions and diagnostic criteria have been reproduced from the Diagnostics and Statistical Manual of Mental Disorders, Fourth edition, with permission.

20.3.) INFANCY, CHILDHOOD, ADOLESCENCE

A) DISORDERS RESULTING IN POOR SCHOOL PERFORMANCE:

mental retardation	• **IQ < 70** (2 standard deviations below norm) • onset before 18 years o in most cases cause remains unknown
autistic disorder [1]	o more common in boys than girls • impaired social interaction • impaired communication • stereotypic behavior
dyslexia	• difficulty with spelling and reading • comprehension of spoken language is intact o has strong genetic link
ADHD	o more common in males • at least for 6 months • at least 2 settings, e.g. home and school • significant impairment in social or academic functioning o may be predominant **inattentive type** o may be predominant **hyperactive type** impulsiveness and poor social skills often persist into adulthood

[1] *may have amazing special skills (mathematics)…*

330

B) <u>DISORDERS RELATED TO "GROWING UP"</u>:

enuresis	<ul><li>age at least **5 years**</li><li>significant distress</li><li>exclude drugs, medical conditions</li></ul>
encopresis	<ul><li>age at least **4 years**</li><li>exclude drugs, medical conditions</li></ul>
separation anxiety	<ul><li>excessive distress when separated from parents, going to school etc.</li><li>onset before 18 years "early onset" if < 6 years of age)</li></ul>

C) <u>RARE DISORDERS</u>:

Asperger's disorder	<ul><li>like autistic disorder **without impairment in language** or cognitive development</li></ul>
Rett's disorder	<ul><li>normal development first 5 months</li><li>then: **decelerated head growth**, loss of previously acquired skills, severe psychomotor retardation</li></ul>
Tourette's disorder	<ul><li>**motor and vocal tics**</li><li>onset before age 18 years</li><li>duration at least 1 year</li></ul>

331

20.4.) <u>PERSONALITY DISORDERS - 1</u>

<u>GENERAL CRITERIA:</u>

(1.) pattern is inflexible across a broad range of situations
(2.) pattern of experience or behavior markedly deviant from cultural norms
(3.) significant distress and impairment of functioning

paranoid	• distrusting, suspicious
schizoid	• socially detached • **neither desires nor enjoys close relationships** • indifferent to praise or criticism
schizotypal	• **eccentric behavior** • odd or magical beliefs • unusual perceptions • inappropriate affect

20.5.) <u>PERSONALITY DISORDERS - 2</u>

antisocial	<ul><li>**disregards for rights of others**</li><li>reckless, impulsive, irritable</li></ul>
borderline	<ul><li>**intense but highly unstable relationships**</li><li>identity disturbance</li><li>self-damaging behavior, suicidal</li><li>paranoid ideations</li><li>dissociative symptoms</li></ul>
histrionic	<ul><li>excessively emotional</li><li>**needs to be center of attention**</li></ul>
narcissistic	<ul><li>**sense of grandiosity and self-importance**</li><li>sense of entitlement → envy</li><li>lack of empathy → arrogant behavior</li></ul>

20.6.) PERSONALITY DISORDERS - 3

obsessive-compulsive	• **sense of perfection that interferes with task completion** • preoccupied with details, rules etc. • unable to discard • unable to delegate • rigid, stubborn
avoidant	• social inhibition • **fear of shame or ridicule** • views self as inferior
dependent	• submissive, clinging behavior • difficulty making decisions without reassurance • **feels helpless**

20.7.) AMNESIA

You must distinguish organic from psychological causes:

ORGANIC	PSYCHOLOGICAL
• remote memory intact	• mixture of recent and remote
• emotional events remembered	• emotional events forgotten
• anterograde and retrograde amnesia	• only retrograde amnesia

20.8.) <u>COGNITIVE DISORDERS</u>

Clinically significant deficit in cognition and memory.
Caused either by a general medical condition or chemicals (drugs, toxins).

delirium	• disturbance of consciousness • disturbance of cognition (memory, orientation, language) • rapid onset, fluctuating • usually due to medical conditions or drugs
dementia	• no disturbance of consciousness • disturbance of cognition (memory, orientation, language) • gradual onset
Alzheimer dementia	**exclude:** Parkinson, Huntington, brain tumor, cerebrovascular diseases, hypothyroidism, vit. B12 or folic acid deficiency, HIV infection etc.
vascular dementia	• suggested if dementia plus focal signs • step-like (rather than gradual) decline

Especially in elderly patients it is important not to mistake depression for dementia!
This may help you to distinguish:

	DEMENTIA	DEPRESSION
insight	- absent	- present
recall of famous persons	- absent	- present
vegetative signs	- rare	- insomnia - constipation - anorexia

20.9.) <u>SCHIZOPHRENIA: HISTORICAL CRITERIA</u>

Emil Kraepelin	• "dementia precox" (cognitive process, early onset)
Eugen Bleuler	• "schizophrenia" • schism between thoughts, emotions and behavior o not split personality!
Bleuler's four A	A ssociations (loose) A ffect inappropriateness A utism A mbivalence
Kurt Schneider	<u>First rank symptoms</u>: • audible thoughts • arguing, discussing or commenting voices • somatic passivity experiences • thought withdrawal • thought broadcasting • delusions

Occasionally, patients may have schizophrenia without showing any of Kurt Schneider's first rank symptoms.

20.10.) SCHIZOPHRENIA: MODERN CRITERIA

diagnostic criteria	• **duration at least 6 months** [1] • active phase at least 1 month (unless treated) • must exclude drugs or medical condition!
positive symptoms	• delusions • hallucinations
negative symptoms	• flat affect • alogia • avolition
subtypes	➤ paranoid ➤ catatonic ➤ disorganized
good prognostic features	• good premorbid functioning • short prodromal phase • absence of blunted or flat affect

[1] *includes prodromal, active and residual phase*

(1.) **Schizoid** personality disorder is unrelated to schizophrenia.

(2.) **Schizotypal** personality disorder is regarded to be the premorbid personality type of many schizophrenics.

(3.) However, most persons with schizotypal personality <u>do not</u> develop schizophrenia.

Family with high level of expressed emotions increases the probability of a relapse in a schizophrenic patient.

20.11.) <u>SCHIZOPHRENIFORM</u>

Criteria for diagnosis of schizophrenia are very strict. If not exactly fulfilled, you must make one of the following diagnoses instead:

schizophreniform disorder	• like schizophrenia • duration **< 6 months**
brief psychotic disorder	• like schizophrenia • duration **< 1 month**
schizoaffective disorder	• major depressive, manic or mixed episode concurrent with symptoms of schizophrenia • **delusions or hallucinations for 2 weeks in absence of prominent mood symptoms** [1]
delusional disorder	• **non-bizarre** delusions [2] • criteria for schizophrenia never been met
substance-induced psychotic disorder	• **alcohol, hallucinogens, cocaine, PCP...** • prominent delusions or hallucinations • absence of intact reality testing • does not occur exclusively during the drug induced delirium

[1] *if delusions and hallucinations occur only during the depressive (or manic) phase it should be classified as **major depressive disorder (or bipolar disorder) with psychotic features!***

[2] *real life situations such as being followed, poisoned, loved and deceived, etc...*

20.12.) <u>MOOD DISORDERS - EPISODES</u>

Mood episodes are components of mood disorders and cannot be diagnosed as
separate entities, but you need to know the criteria for episodes in order to diagnose
a mood disorder properly!

major depressive episode	<ul><li>depressed mood</li><li>diminished interest</li><li>weight loss</li><li>early morning insomnia</li><li>feeling of worthlessness</li></ul><ul><li>o **do not diagnose this within 2 months of bereavement !**</li></ul>
manic episode	<ul><li>decreased need for sleep</li><li>talkative, flight of ideas</li><li>goal directed but very distractible</li><li>**marked impairment of social or occupational functioning**</li></ul>
hypomanic episode	<ul><li>markedly elevated mood</li><li>uncharacteristic change in behavior</li><li>**not severe enough to impair social or occupational functioning**</li><li>duration > 4 days</li></ul>

20.13.) <u>MOOD DISORDERS - ENTITIES</u>

Mood disorders are defined by presence or absence of mood episodes described in (20.12.)

major depressive disorder	• presence of major depressive episode • there has never been a hypomanic, manic or mixed episode • exclude schizophrenia!
bipolar I disorder	• **at least one manic episode**
bipolar II disorder	• at least one major depressive episode and at least one hypomanic episode • **there has never been a manic or mixed episode**
dysthymic disorder	• depressed mood **for > 2 years** • but no major depressive episode
cyclothymic disorder	• numerous hypomanic periods • numerous depressive periods, but no major depressive episode • **for > 2 years**

20.14.) <u>ANXIETY DISORDERS - 1</u>

panic attack	• abrupt onset, peak within 10 min. • palpitations, tachycardia • sweating • trembling, shaking • lightheadedness • fear of dying **Derealization:** feeling of unreality of the external world **Depersonalization:** feeling of being detached from oneself
agoraphobia	• anxiety of being in **places were a panic attack might occur** and escape would be impossible or embarrassing
panic disorder	• recurrent panic attacks • persistent concern about have additional attacks result in behavioral change • with or without agoraphobia
specific phobia	• persistent excessive fear • cued by presence or anticipation • **patient recognizes that the fear is unrealistic !**
social phobia	• persistent fear of social or performance situations (unfamiliar people, possible scrutiny by others etc.) • **patient recognizes that the fear is unrealistic !**
obsessive-compulsive disorder	**Obsessions:** recurrent thoughts, impulses, images **Compulsions:** repetitive behaviors • **patient recognized at some extent that these are unreasonable**

341

20.15.) <u>ANXIETY DISORDERS - 2</u>

acute stress disorder	• traumatic event → intense fear • dissociative symptoms [1] • dreams, illusions, flashbacks ○ **lasts at least 2 days** ○ **occurs within 4 weeks of event**
posttraumatic stress disorder	• traumatic event → intense fear • dissociative symptoms [1] • dreams, illusions, flashbacks • persistent arousal, hypervigilance ○ **lasts at least 1 month [2]** ○ **occurs any time after event [3]**
generalized anxiety disorder	• excessive worry (work, school etc.) • restlessness, fatigue • irritability, muscle tension • sleep disturbance ○ **duration > 6 months**

[1] *dissociative symptoms:*   *- derealization*
                                      - depersonalization
                                      - sense of numbing, detachment
                                      - absence of emotional responsiveness

[2] *considered "**chronic**" if > 3 months*

[3] *considered "**delayed**" if onset of symptoms > 6 months after event*

20.16.) <u>SOMATOFORM DISORDERS</u>

Patients present with physical symptoms that cannot be fully explained by a general medical condition (axis III).

A) <u>UNINTENTIONAL (INVOLUNTARY)</u>:

somatization (Briquet's syndrome)	• **sickly for most of life** • GI, reproductive, cardiopulmonary, pain etc. • diagnosed, when at least 12 symptoms are present and history of several years.
conversion disorder (hysterical neurosis)	• **"pseudoneurological"** symptoms: (blindness, paresthesia, paralysis…) • symptoms begin and end suddenly • often misdiagnosed as "malingering"
hypochondriasis	• **unrealistic interpretation** of body signs • belief to have serious disease that goes unrecognized by family and physicians

B) <u>INTENTIONAL (VOLUNTARY)</u>:

factitious disorder	• intentional feigning of symptoms • **motivation: to assume the "sick role"** • external incentives (economic gain, avoiding legal responsibilities etc.) are absent !
malingering	• intentional feigning of symptoms • **motivation: economic gain, avoiding legal responsibilities...**

20.17.) <u>DISSOCIATIVE DISORDERS</u>

One of the functions of the "ego" is to integrate consciousness, memory and experiences to form an identity. Breakdown of this integration results in dissociative disorders which usually are sudden and transient, but also may be chronic.

dissociative amnesia	• **inability to recall important personal information** • goes beyond forgetfulness
dissociative fugue	• sudden, unexpected travel away from home • **inability to recall one's past** • **assume new identity**
depersonalization	• **feeling like one is in a dream** • feeling detached from oneself • reality testing remains intact during this experience
dissociative identity disorder (multiple personality disorder)	• **two or more distinct personalities** recurrently taking control of person's behavior • inability to recall important personal information

*In order to make a diagnosis of dissociative disorder, other causes of amnesia, fugue or depersonalization such as **trauma, drug abuse, acute stress disorder, posttraumatic stress disorder etc. must be excluded.***

Despite the popular notion to the contrary, multiple personality disorder is completely distinct from schizophrenia.

20.18.) <u>EATING DISORDERS</u>

Excessive emphasis on body-shape and weight for self-evaluation and self-esteem. Depressive symptoms and obsessive-compulsive features are common.

ANOREXIA NERVOSA	BULIMIA
• **refusal to maintain weight** (>15% below normal)	• **recurrent episodes of binge eating** • lack of control over eating behavior
• intense fear of becoming fat • disturbed body image	• persistent concern about body weight
• amenorrhea	• self-induced vomiting [1] • abuse of laxatives, diuretics
	• patients are ashamed of their eating behavior and try to conceal

[1] *look for teeth erosions due to gastric acid!*

Obesity is NOT an eating-disorder and should be coded as general medical condition (axis III).

20.19.) ANTIPSYCHOTICS - SIDE EFFECTS

ACUTE DYSTONIA

occurs within hours of medication (most common with high-potency IM use)
- Torticollis, jaw dislocation, tongue protrusion
- Usually disappears eventually (tolerance)
- ➤ Switch to another antipsychotic (thioridazine)
- ➤ Give anticholinergics

AKATHISIA

may occur at any time
- Feeling of muscular discomfort
- Relentless movements, sit, stand, sit, stand...
- ➤ Reduce dosage!

PARKINSONISM

occurs within weeks to months of treatment
- Muscle stiffness: cogwheel rigidity
- Shuffling, drooling
- Usually disappears eventually (tolerance)
- ➤ Add anticholinergics for several weeks

TARDIVE DYSKINESIA

occurs after many months of treatment
- Choreoathetosis, tongue protrusion, lateral movements of jaw
- Most mild cases eventually remit but more severe ones are often irreversible
- ➤ Reduce dosage, switch or stop

MALIGNANT SYNDROME

high fever, heart rate and blood pressure
- Muscle rigidity
- ➤ Immediately discontinue drug!
- ➤ Cool patient, give dantrolene and anti-Parkinson

20.20.) <u>ANTIDEPRESSANTS - SIDE EFFECTS</u>

SEROTONIN SELECTIVE REUPTAKE INHIBITORS
- decreased libido
- insomnia, restlessness, decreased appetite

TRICYCLIC ANTIDEPRESSANTS
- Anticholinergic action: - blurred vision
  - dry mouth,
  - constipation
  - urinary retention
- Sedation
- **ECG:** prolonged PQ, depressed ST
  (tricyclics are contraindicated in patients with AV conduction defect)

MAO INHIBITORS
- Orthostatic hypotension
- Weight gain, edema
- ➤ Avoid beer, wine, cheese, fresh oranges...
  (tyramine induced hypertensive crisis)

LITHIUM
- Tremors
- Nausea, vomiting, diarrhea
- Confusion
- Convulsions

- ➤ If signs of toxicity (coarse tremors and ataxia) develop:
  - treat as medical emergency!

 Never ever combine several antidepressants!

ABBREVIATIONS

a/w	associated with	IBD	inflammatory bowel disease
ACE	angiotensin converting enzyme	IC	inspiratory capacity
AFP	alpha-fetoprotein	ITP	idiopathic thrombocytopenic purpura
AGA	appropriate for gestational age	IUD	intrauterine device
ANA	antinuclear antigen	IVF	in vitro fertilization
ANCA	antineutrophil cytoplasmic antibody	L.M.	light microscope
ARDS	acute respiratory distress syndrome	LAD	left ascending coronary artery
ARF	acute renal failure	LBBB	left bundle branch block
ASD	atrial septal defect	LDL	low density lipoproteins
ATN	acute tubular necrosis	LES	lower esophageal sphincter
BMI	body mass index	LGA	large for gestational age
CEA	carcinoembryonic antigen	LMP	last menstrual period
CHD	coronary heart disease	LSD	lysergic acid diethylamine
CHF	congestive heart failure	MAO	monoamine oxidase
COPD	chronic obstructive pulmonary disease	MCH	mean corpuscular hemoglobin
		MCHC	mean corpuscular hemoglobin concentration
CRFLX	circumflex coronary artery		
CSF	cerebrospinal fluid	MCV	mean corpuscular volume
CXR	chest x-ray	MI	myocardial infarction
DHEA	dehydroepiandrosterone	MMR	measles-mumps-rubella
DIC	disseminated intravascular coagulation	MS	multiple sclerosis
		NBT	nitroblue tetrazolium
DIP	distal interphalangeal joint	NIDDM	non-insulin-dependent diabetes mellitus
DM	diabetes mellitus	NSAID	non-steroidal antiinflammatory drug
DTP	diphtheria-tetanus-pertussis	PAS	periodic acid Schiff
DUI	driving under the influence	PCP	phencyclidine
DCT	deep vein thrombosis	PDA	patent ductus arteriosus
E.M.	electron microscope	PEEP	positive end-expiratory pressure
ECV	extracellular volume	PIP	proximal interphalangeal joint
ENA	extractable nuclear antigen	PMN	polymorphonuclear leukocyte
ERCP	endoscopic retrograde cholangiopancreatography	PPD	purified protein derivative
		PSA	prostate specific antigen
ERV	expiratory reserve volume	PT	prothrombin time
FTA	fluorescent treponemal antibody	PTH	parathormone
G6PD	glucose-6-phosphate dehydrogenase	PTT	partial thromboplastin time
GBM	glomerular basement membrane	RA	rheumatoid arthritis
GFR	glomerular filtration rate	RBBB	right bundle branch block
GN	glomerulonephritis	RBC	red blood cell
hCG	human chorionic gonadotropin	RCA	right coronary artery
HDL	high density lipoproteins	RFLP	restriction fragment length polymorphism
HLA	human leukocytic antigen	RV	residual volume

349

SGA	small for gestational age	TLC	total lung capacity
SIADH	syndrome of inappropriate ADH	TTP	thrombotic thrombocytopenic purpura
SIDS	sudden infant death syndrome	UMN	upper motor neuron
SLE	systemic lupus erythematosus	UTI	urinary tract infection
SS	systemic sclerosis	VC	vital capacity
STDs	sexually transmitted diseases	VDRL	Venereal Disease Research Laboratories
Tb	tuberculosis	VIP	vasoactive intestinal peptide
TBG	thyroxin binding globulin	VLDL	very low density lipoproteins
TC	total cholesterol	VSD	ventricular septal defect
TG	triglyceride	WBC	white blood cell
TIA	transient ischemic attack		

INDEX

358

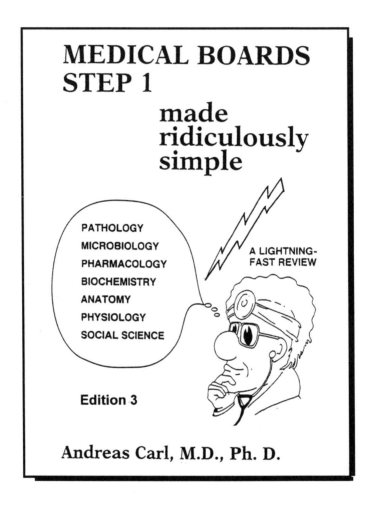

MEDICAL BOARDS
STEP 1

made
ridiculously
simple

PATHOLOGY

MICROBIOLOGY

PHARMACOLOGY

BIOCHEMISTRY

ANATOMY

PHYSIOLOGY

SOCIAL SCIENCE

A LIGHTNING-
FAST REVIEW

Edition 3

Andreas Carl, M.D., Ph. D.

368 pages   -   333 charts

◆ All the facts about Basic Medical Sciences in chart format.

◆ With clinical correlations.

MEDICAL BOARDS STEP 3

made ridiculously simple

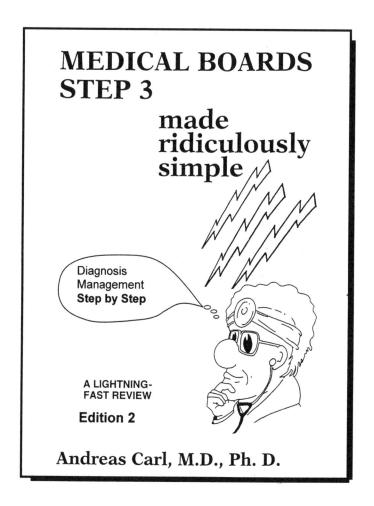

Diagnosis
Management
Step by Step

**A LIGHTNING-
FAST REVIEW**

Edition 2

Andreas Carl, M.D., Ph. D.

312 pages - 395 charts

♦ A Step-by-Step Approach (*"what to do next ?"*)

♦ Diagnosis and Management of Diseases